Secrets to living
longer & feeling fantastic

2 WEEKS TO A YOUNGER YOU

gabriela peacock

An Hachette UK Company
www.hachette.co.uk

First published in Great Britain in 2023 by
Kyle Books, an imprint of Octopus Publishing Group Limited
Carmelite House, 50 Victoria Embankment
London EC4Y 0DZ
www.kylebooks.co.uk

ISBN: 978 1 91423 990 8

Distributed in the US by Hachette Book Group, 1290 Avenue of the Americas,
4th and 5th Floors, New York, NY 10104

Distributed in Canada by Canadian Manda Group, 664 Annette St., Toronto, Ontario,
Canada M6S 2C8

Publishing Director: Judith Hannam
Publisher: Joanna Copestick
Project Editor: Isabel Jessop
Design: Nikki Dupin at Studio Nic & Lou
Writer: Clare Bennett
Copy-editor: Claire Rogers
Lifestyle photography: Kate Martin
Food photography: Kate Whitaker
Production: Lucy Carter and Nic Jones

A Cataloguing in Publication record for this title is available from the British Library.

Printed and bound in China.

10 9 8 7 6 5 4 3 2 1

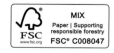

Gabriela Peacock qualified as a Nutritional Therapist with BSc (Hons) in Health Science from the University of Westminster
and has a diploma in Naturopathic Nutrition. She set up her first clinic in Belgravia in 2012. Gabriela's work focuses
on achieving optimum health through a realistic approach to modern life. In 2016, she founded GP Nutrition, launching
her own range of specialised supplement programmes and is regularly featured in the press and on TV. Gabriela lives in
west London with her husband and three children.

contents

let's get started

Welcome to my second book! This time around we are talking about longevity – one of the most progressive areas in science and nutrition. This first section will help you understand what makes us age and how we can radically influence that process. Because knowledge is the foundation from which you can change anything – including the future you...

1

do you know how amazing you are?

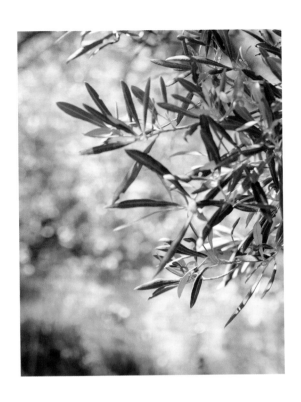

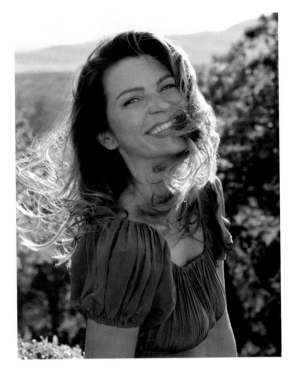

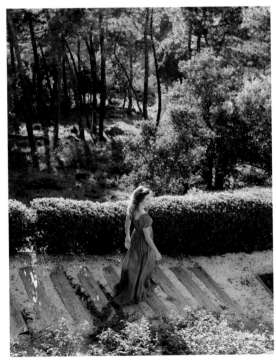

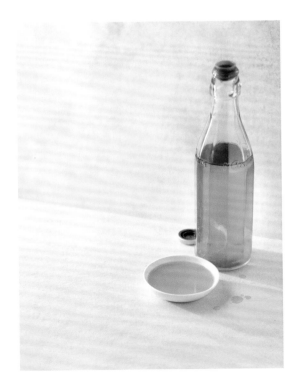

do you know how amazing you are?

Let's get one thing straight. You are absolutely amazing. You are more complex than anything NASA could ever dream of creating, times a billion. You are unique, mysterious, intelligent beyond comprehension and – if I may just show-off on your behalf (and mine, come to think of it) – most of that brilliance is effortless. If you had any real idea about the number of jobs, decisions and successful problem-solving tasks your body undertakes every moment you are alive, your head might explode. Except it wouldn't because your inner mechanisms are way too sophisticated to do something as stupid as that.

The human body is a construct of extraordinary magnificence. Incredible things happen in you all the time without you even realising. The whole of your skin replaces itself every single month. Your nose is believed to be capable of identifying a trillion different scents. In the space of a single second, your body produces 25 million cells. All this and you might just be drinking a cup of tea, scrolling through Instagram or staring at a wall. What your body does without any active input from you is quite simply breath-taking.

When it comes to ageing, the preconception is that it's something to fear. That life gets worse. That we look worse and we feel worse – but does that have to be true? Ageing is a completely natural process, but our fears are driven by the notion of physical and mental decline – and this is not without some foundation. So what if we knew of a way to make ourselves feel and look fantastic as we age? To know that we would have energy, a strong immune system and mental clarity and still look like a million bucks might completely change our relationship with ageing. The science around longevity is starting to do just that.

Spoiler alert

We all age. So why not make it work for us? I mean, *really* make it work for us. For centuries, humankind has been searching for the fountain of youth (where is it?) – from Cleopatra bathing in asses' milk to keep her skin supple and youthful, to Dorian Gray selling his soul to preserve his beauty as his portrait decays in the attic (you can see why he went there – it might have worked) – and we have long considered ageing as something to ward off. The good news is: this book will empower you to redefine what ageing means to you. You won't even have to make a pact with a malignant force or spend hours milking a donkey every time you want a bath.

what makes us scared to age?

Our relationship with ageing probably begins with the fear of how our looks will change. We associate looking young with feeling young and being young, as if that is the only way in which we can remain a contender in life. We think that if we are able to keep ourselves looking as young as possible, we'll manage to slow our ageing down and make it go away. This is particularly true for women, whose sense of self-worth and attractiveness has long been associated with youth, while the idea of male ageing leans more into status and experience. Who decided that was how it should work?

Let's think about this for a moment. Do you really want to *be* 20 or do you want to just *look* 20? Being 20 has many charms – but so does having your own home, having a successful career and not having to ask your dad to pick you up from a nightclub at 4am because you're drunk and no Uber will go near you. To age is to live. To experience life in all its many colours. We should embrace it, not do everything we can to get out of it (like a school WhatsApp group).

How do we choose to frame these completely natural phases of our lives? It comes down to where we set the baseline for what makes us happy and content in life, from our relationship with food to how we perceive ourselves through our many physical changes. We might look at the fine lines forming around our eyes as the beginning of physical deterioration – or we might feel they represent everything that has made us laugh over the years. We get to decide.

What would life be like if no one mentioned how old they were ever again? Pretty liberating. The human race is a bit too over-enthusiastic in placing meaning in numbers. We stand on a set of scales and judge ourselves for the number we see between our feet. We stare at the tiny numbered square in our clothes and wish it were lower. Anyone (anyone??) who has read my first book will know I am closed for business when it comes to any kind of number- or judgement-related approach to our sense of self. I'd rather be having a good time, thanks for asking.

looking to the future

The fact is, human beings are living longer than ever, so our conversation around ageing needs to change. How do we make it work for us? Because the chances are, we will be around for quite some time. Latest research predicts that by 2050, the number of people in the world aged over 60 will double to more than 2 billion, while the number of people aged over 80 will triple to reach around 400 million. While progressions in science and medicine are playing a significant role in this, we need to make it clear that the aim is not to be kept alive for years on end if quality of life is diminished, but to truly live and feel great for as long as possible. That sounds like a plan.

It's exciting that the science around longevity is changing the entire landscape of how ageing has traditionally been considered. We are learning so much about what happens to the body as it progresses through the years and what we can do to influence it so that we look and feel fantastic. Turns out it's A LOT.

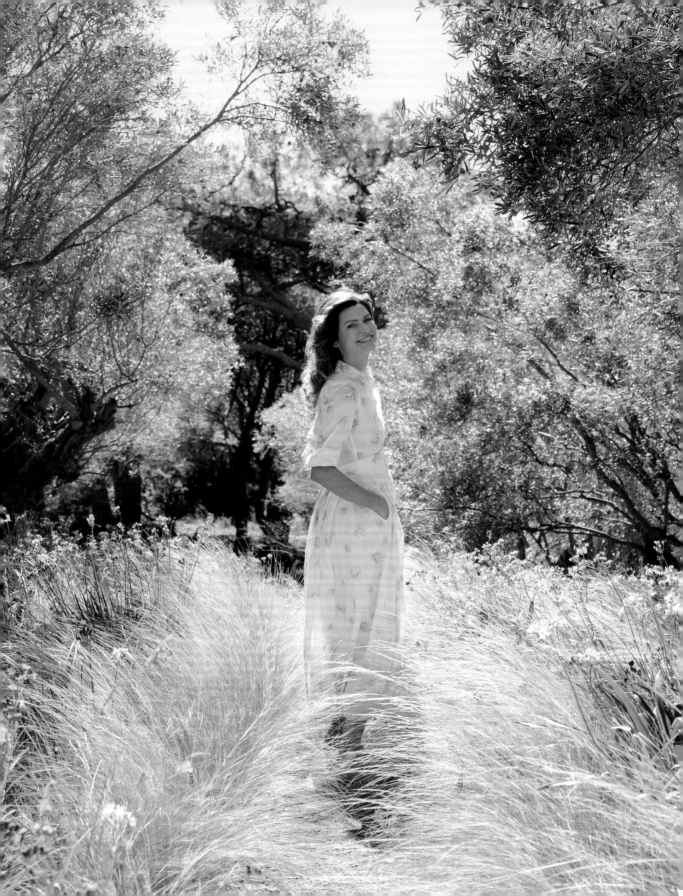

2

the science
of ageing

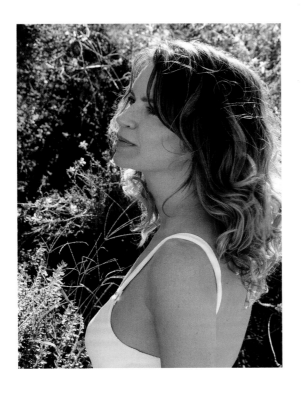
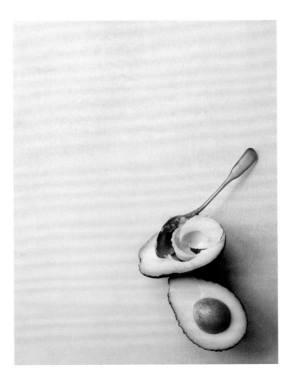
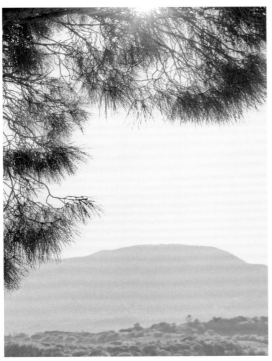
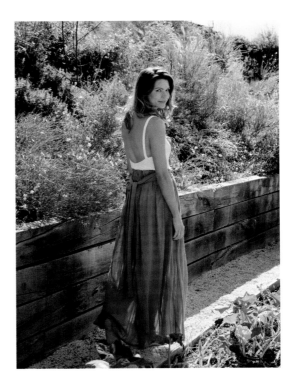

the one and only you

Human beings are all about cells – and yet cells are not actually alive. They are like storage containers for information that makes us who we are. This information is our DNA, and while the DNA of most human beings is 99.9 per cent identical, that difference makes *all* the difference. It makes your DNA the entirely exclusive, one-off instruction manual of you.

DNA appears as two chains that form a spiral-shaped ladder, which is organised into genes within chromosomes – collectively called genomes. Genes form codes that instruct cells to make proteins, the building blocks of the body, which in turn make enzymes, antibodies, hormones, haemoglobin and other critical components that form a living human. Genes carry information passed down from thousands of years of ancestors and have the potential to keep going and going through descendants long after someone has left this earth.

Aside from proteins, each cell houses other essential ingredients, like mitochondria and the nucleus, and together with the essential seasoning that is the mystery of life, they form the miracle that is you. Living, breathing, thinking, feeling, remembering, eating, digesting, sleeping, weeping, laughing, sulking, compassionate, selfish, complicated, glorious you.

the sometimes thankless job of looking after you

The cells of the body work day and night – with no duvet days – to rebalance, manage, organise and fix everything thrown at them. At the end of it, in spite of their efforts, they are rewarded with death. There's always a younger cell after their job. It was ever thus.

None of us has any idea of the sheer scale of work that goes on beneath the surface of our bodies. Take liver cells, for example. Our liver performs around 500 jobs on a daily basis, which includes clearing out all the chemicals you come into contact with. That might begin as soon as you're in the shower in the morning, washing yourself with a product containing parabens, which get into your system via your skin and have to be processed out again through the liver.

We do horrible things to ourselves all the time. Some are obvious, like eating processed food, smoking cigarettes, drinking alcohol; and some less so, like serving food cooked in non-stick pans, inhaling city pollutants and drinking water from plastic bottles. Our bodies take on each task as best they can without any knowledge or conscious contribution from us.

Then there are our immune cells. Our own private army on constant alert to keep us safe from pathogens. You might be doing something as innocuous as walking down the street, breathing in and out – but inside, it is full-blown action stations for your immune cells, as they furiously work against time to clear out the pollutants entering your body through your lungs and skin before they harm you. It's like a never-ending episode of *Homeland* with no advert breaks, and yet, for the most part, even when it's being hammered from all sides, your body will find its centre ground again.

We survive so much without realising we're surviving anything. Every single day. That makes us worth looking after, doesn't it? With this tiny insight into what our bodies are capable of without us even trying, imagine what they could do with our help. If we choose to step up and take part in our body's daily efforts to keep us upright and alive, we have the potential to completely reshape our future. We can harness our own innate power and move through life healthy, happy and ageing not just gracefully, but magnificently.

what is ageing?

So! What makes us age? Well, needless to say, there is no single answer – more like a whole set of answers all holding hands and giving each other side eye. As we know, within the body nothing works in isolation, and ageing is no exception.

Scientific research on the subject of ageing continues to evolve, of course, but at the moment, nine processes have been identified that lead to changes associated with the signs of ageing. Some are mysterious; all are complex – but they happen to varying degrees in all of us.

Many people tend to think of ageing as simply genetic, therefore there's not much we can do about it and, oh well. But studies keep showing how much our environment and the choices we make in everyday life impact these processes in very profound ways. This means we need to take action before there's a problem – prevention is like a pension for your health. It pays dividends in the end.

We have more autonomy over how we age than we might have first thought... Game-changing autonomy. Bear this in mind as we take a closer look at the nine hallmarks of ageing – and don't start crying, because we have cunning plans up our sleeve to make you feel better than you ever imagined.

chronological age vs biological age

Your chronological age is the number of years since you were born. Your biological age is how old your body seems, based on a number of factors, including how your chromosomes have changed over time. Chronological age, you can do nothing about – but biological age, you can – and that's the one that counts.

when DNA is under fire
(AKA genomic instability)

Let's start with DNA. DNA is the set of unique instructions that dictate how your entire body develops, behaves and functions. Half of these design plans are inherited from your mother and half from your father. They are extremely precious and the body needs to protect them (we could be pitching for a thrilling action film here).

But like all interesting things in life, there is obviously an element of jeopardy just to keep things spicy. DNA is constantly under assault on an enormous scale from things like pollutants, UV rays, free radicals and pesticides, which all want to bring it down. Therefore, the body works hard to keep DNA safe.

Think of DNA like a metaphorical record collection. Each area of the body stores its DNA (the songs) in genes (the record), which are kept within chromosomes (the record sleeve) within cells (a record storage box) and then organised into genomes (the music genre).

DNA is not helpless, though – it knows how to repair itself. But that said, its capabilities are limited and its attempts to repair can sometimes result in mutations. As we age, the increased daily battering it takes starts to wear it down, resulting in what is known as genomic instability.

You can be exemplary in how you take care of your record collection, but eventually, the records will inevitably become scratched, the sound quality will diminish and the sleeves will end up scuffed as the years roll by because that's just life. It's the same with the genomes in the body as it ages. Think of that next time you're playing one of your favourite old Duran Duran records and wondering why the needle is now jumping a bit.

when things start to unravel
(AKA telomere attrition)

Telomeres are caps that sit on the end of a chromosome like a bottle top. As cells divide to replace old dead cells, an essential process to keep the body functioning efficiently, a little part of the telomere is lost until eventually none is left. This results in cells not being able to divide – which leads to ageing – a process known as telomere attrition.

Understanding the life span of the telomere can help predict a person's life span. Yes, telomeres are kind of a big deal – and that's putting it mildly. Studying them has revolutionised our understanding of chronology's role in the ageing process. All this from just a little deteriorating cap.

when the captain goes AWOL
(AKA epigenetic alterations)

Epigenomes are groups of chemical compounds responsible for activating genes. They tell genes what to do, where to do it and when to do it. Once the genes have received their instructions from the epigenomes, the DNA stored within those genes informs how these instructions are interpreted.

The relationship between epigenomes and genes is essential and what affects one affects the other. The passage of time, environmental factors, illness and disease start to take their toll on epigenomes and this makes them less effective, which impacts gene expression. A ship needs a captain to steer it or the crew will just get lazy and drink rum all day.

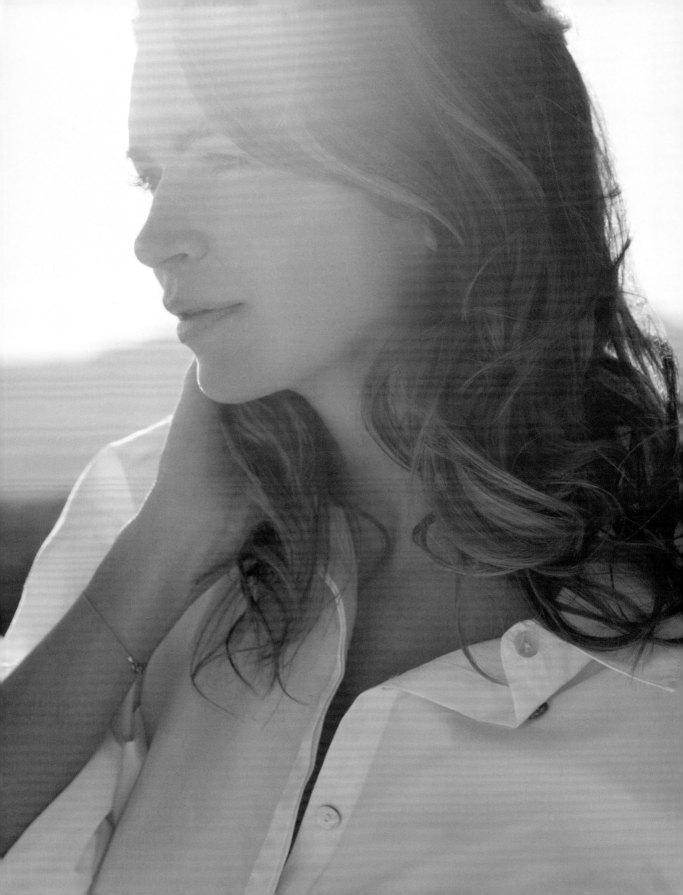

When the building falls into disrepair
(AKA loss of proteostasis)

How to put this? Proteins are EVERYTHING. They are the body's building blocks. They're essential to the production and repair of cells, as well as chemical reactions within the body. Proteins are what make you work.

Proteostasis ('protein' and 'stasis', which means balance) is completely vital for health and harmony within the body. Imagine proteins as the bricks and mortar of a building. If they are not maintained properly, and if damage is not addressed or replacements made where necessary, the building will fall into disrepair.

If proteostasis stops running smoothly, everything takes a hit. It can be caused by a lack of antioxidants allowing free radicals to run riot or environmental stressors – and this can cause chaos. It's like trying to rebuild a house with not enough – and badly made – bricks.

when the look outs stop noticing things
(AKA deregulated nutrient sensing)

Nutrients in food are vital in helping the body's cells do their job. When food is ingested, nutrient sensors on cells detect the released nutrients and use them to turn food into energy – the chemical reaction known as metabolism.

Nutrient sensors have a complicated job on their hands, though. They don't know when or what you're going to eat so they have to constantly make decisions about how many nutrients to use at any given time.

The process of metabolism has its side effects – it produces free radicals, the pirates of the molecule world. They roam around the body with one electron when they should have two, looking to snatch the missing half of the pair from another cell, leaving it dead or damaged. It's normal for the body to have some free radicals mugging other cells, but things can go too far and this is known as oxidative stress.

This in turn impacts how nutrient sensors are able to detect nutrients in food. Damaged by oxidative stress as time passes, they become confused, making them less able to detect nutrient availability, which can age cells.

when the batteries start failing
(AKA mitochondrial dysfunction)

It seems like getting older and feeling tired go hand in hand. There are two reasons for this. First, free radicals cause damage, triggered by unhealthy choices like smoking, drinking or having a poor diet. Second, the body can get tricked into thinking it doesn't need to produce much energy. To understand why this happens, we need to go to the power source.

Ninety per cent of the body's energy comes from mitochondria, the batteries of cells. Their main job is to charge up their cells in order to support the body's metabolism. However, mitochondria also produce free radicals, which, of course, will try to steal electrons. Rude.

The ageing process slows down the production of mitochondria, which puts pressure on what already exists. Overworked and underpaid, they struggle to produce energy and this makes the body feel tired.

However, what's interesting about mitochondria is that they respond to the body's energy demands. If a person sits around not using up much energy, the mitochondria don't feel they need to produce much. However, if they're active, mitochondria will raise their game and produce more energy to keep up. Physical activity may take energy, but it also produces energy, and this is extremely significant when it comes to longevity.

when the workforce goes rogue
(AKA cellular senescence)

A cell's ability to divide is crucial for it to fulfil its role within the body. When it can no longer perform this function, the cell becomes damaged and effectively stops turning up to work. This is known as cellular senescence. This perfectly natural process is actually a form of protection, as it prevents these zombie cells from multiplying and remaining active enough to cause problems.

The body is normally able to produce more functioning cells to make up for those that become senescent, but as we age, this cell production slows down and the number of senescent cells increases. For example, the reason why skin starts to wrinkle and sag as we age is that skin cells stop renewing due to cellular senescence. Cellular senescence can also deplete the body's ability to repair damaged tissue and inflammation, which are major contributors to ageing. They are the old tins at the back of the cupboard from ten years ago that need throwing out.

when the old guard won't retire
(AKA stem cell exhaustion)

Cells are instructed by epigenomes to carry out a job within the body. Once that job has been accepted – lung cell, muscle cell, brain cell, kidney cell – they stick to it for life.

The only exception to this rule are stem cells. They're like supreme athletes who could turn their hand to any sport.

Stem cells are able to respond to the body's needs by assigning themselves a job to support the production and function of new cells all over the body, showing up to an area that needs reinforcements and adapting accordingly. Their work is crucial if things are to run smoothly, but ageing means that stem cells start to become tired. The knock-on effect can result in fewer new cells being produced and the older cells starting to outnumber them. This is known as stem cell exhaustion. I want to lie down just thinking about it.

when cells stop talking
(AKA altered intercellular communication)

If there's one thing cells love, it's to talk. They chat to each other all day through a complex system of chemical signals in order to manage and maintain the body's ever changing needs. As the body begins to age, this giant cell WhatsApp group starts to break down. Cells stop responding to texts, voice notes are muffled and they start leaving their groups in droves. This is known as altered intercellular communication.

Why does this happen? One of the main causes is inflammation. This key immune response is designed to protect and flush out damaged areas or to fight off infection. But what usually works as part of an acute response can sometimes overstay its welcome and start to damage perfectly healthy cells. Senescent cells should also be looking a bit guilty right about now. That's because they release chemicals that contribute to inflammation and exacerbate the problem. AND they are capable of hacking into the healthy cell WhatsApp group and encouraging them to become senescent, too.

So what is the difference between genetics and epigenetics?

A brief recap. Genetics is the DNA information you inherit from your parents that determines how your body functions and develops. This happens when epigenomes issue orders to proteins, the body's building blocks, telling them how the DNA within the body's genes would like them to behave.

Epigenetics is the study of how environment and lifestyle impact the way in which genes are expressed. These influences include everything from nutrition to sleeping habits, cognitive function, life events, sense of community and emotional well-being. Epigenetics is like an artist and DNA is the palette of paints. The artist is given one palette of paints to work with, but they get to decide which ones they want to use.

Diet, pollutants, exercise, lifestyle choices and significant experiences can all lead to epigenetic modifications, i.e. how the artist uses the paints – that's why identical twins separated at birth, but who share the same DNA, can go on to develop differently, whether that be through variations in weight, health or life span.

What all this means is that epigenetics can be influenced and this will ultimately have a profound effect on the body and how it progresses through life. DNA inherited from your parents and influenced by the environment you grew up in (like bad diets, lack of exercise or aptitude for weight gain) are not a life sentence. In other words, you have the power to make huge and life-changing alterations to your future self, no matter what you've been through. Heartening news.

There is nothing to be gained in reaching the age of 100 if life isn't good – and that involves more than just not being ill. Having robust health, getting support from family and friends, being active and feeling content and happy will prolong life for the better – especially if life has predominantly followed that pattern for many years. The time to start is now!

blue zones

While chronic disease is prevalent among most ageing populations, there are five parts of the world that seem to buck that trend. Studies have revealed that in these specific areas, elderly people are living long into old age but remaining healthy and active and enjoying life. Known as 'blue zones', these areas have been identified as Ikaria in Greece, Ogliastra in Sardinia, Okinawa in Japan, the Nicoya Peninsula in Costa Rica and the Seventh-day Adventist community in Loma Linda, California.

What do these zones have in common? The answer is diets rich in plant foods, high levels of physical activity and busy social lives (with the occasional glass of red wine thrown in). People are bypassing the negative impacts experienced by so many other elderly populations to live healthily and happily well into their nineties and beyond. They are doing things differently and it shows.

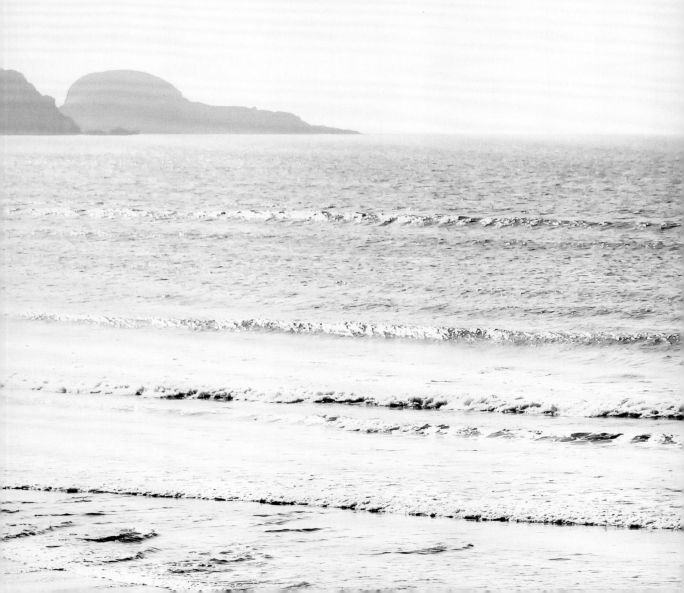

3

the joy
of stress

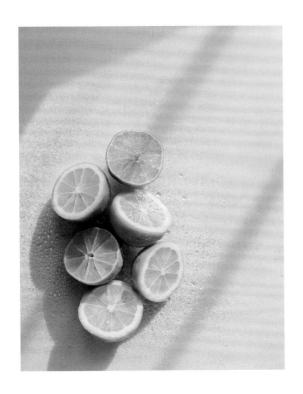
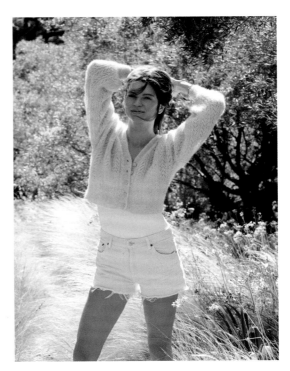
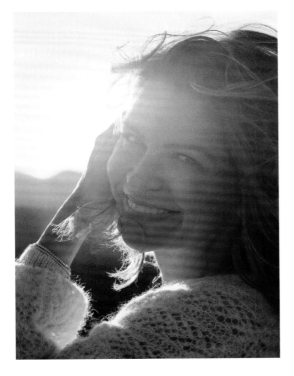
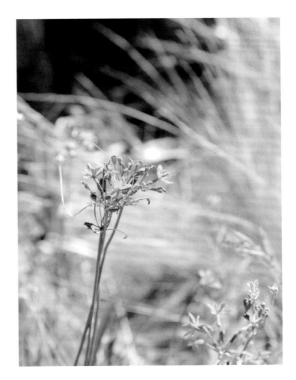

hedonic adaptation:
have we become too comfortable?

Compared to almost all of human existence, life now has never been easier. There are, of course, parts of the world where things are extremely tough and challenging on a daily basis, but in many countries we live very comfortably relative to our ancestors. Perhaps even too comfortably...

Most of human existence has been a pretty rough ride. Even a generation as recent as our great-grandparents would marvel at how easy it is to buy the enormous variety of food available to us, to have the access we do to information, travel, heat for our homes and clean water, and to be able to connect with people across the world simply by pressing a few buttons. Life in the modern age has been transformed by the invention of electricity and the progression of medicine, science and technology, enabling many of us to become more interconnected than ever before. And yet, it's not all plain sailing. The absence of so many of the challenges that faced our ancestors has inadvertently created new ones.

A lot of the richest countries in the world are also the most unhealthy. Many of us can have as much of what we want, when we want it – fast food is just an app order away, after all – and this can be harmful not only physically, but also psychologically.

Curiously, humans have long associated success or happiness with excess. Think of ancient Roman nobility gorging on outrageously opulent feasts and making themselves sick using peacock feathers just so they can start all over again. This was considered a sign of wealth and privilege, a marker of social standing – and not just because they loved dormice dipped in honey.

This notion of pleasure-seeking is behind the theory of what is known as hedonic adaptation. Too much of a good thing sets a precarious baseline for what makes a person both physically and mentally happy.

Imagine you've been longing for a new car. The day finally arrives when you get it and you drive it around excitedly, windows down, loudly playing James Blunt on the stereo (or is that just me?). A few weeks down the line and that initial hit will have subsided. Maybe your kids have spilled apple juice all over the back seats and it's covered in dog hair. Your state of euphoria will have settled – in other words, you have adapted to the situation.

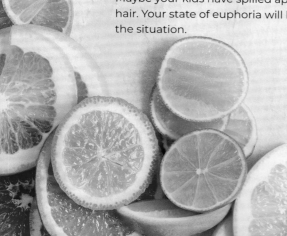

our prehistoric sweet tooth

The same is true with food. We are predisposed to follow the instincts of our neanderthal ancestors, who stocked up on fats, sugars and carbohydrates throughout the seasons because they didn't know where their next food source would come from. The problem now is that the human race has experienced such a disproportionate surge in our evolution that our DNA inheritance has not yet caught up with our modern life of excess. We are effectively living with an 'evolutionary time-lag', which means that in many ways we have become far less resilient than we've ever been.

It's not a coincidence that junk foods tend to be a combination of fats, sugars and carbohydrates. Over time, if you eat these stimulating foods on a regular basis and in large quantities, your body's point of satisfaction becomes too high. You start to need that hit – and in even greater portions. Not only does this create a self-perpetuating craving cycle, but healthy foods simply don't touch the sides when it comes to satiety.

This is because three things are happening. Blood sugar levels are on a rollercoaster – up one minute, down the next – triggering cravings. Constant exposure to sugar means taste buds become physically less able to appreciate something like the taste of a tomato when it's accustomed to the tomato's sugary, very distant relative, ketchup. Plus there is a psychological association: satisfying a physical craving feels good, so we become unable to experience happiness through eating well.

a little note on happiness

It all comes down to where we set the happiness baselines from which we determine what brings us satisfaction. Happiness is a slippery creature. It doesn't exist objectively, which makes it hard to measure. What happiness means will differ from person to person. A group of children from a third-world country may feel heightened feelings of gratitude for food when they have always known it to be scarce, for love when their lives may have faced hardship early on and for school, when getting an education is not a given. Their baseline for happiness may be so low due to the challenges they have faced in life that they experience profound and genuine joy at things many of us in the West are privileged enough to take for granted. In the end, who is happier? A child bursting with excitement because they're allowed to go to school, or a child just back from school, sulking on the sofa because they're allowed to watch YouTube for only an hour?

let's get stressed

Wait. What? Weren't we supposed to be doing everything we could NOT to be stressed? What's going on?

You might not like the sound of this, but the reality is that we are biologically designed to survive in conditions that are far more challenging than the ones we live in.

The world has become fixated with stress. We talk about it, we experience it, we do everything we can to alleviate it – but is there an argument that stress under the right circumstances can actually bring its own form of growth? There is a well-researched scientific hypothesis that we under-challenge ourselves. We wrap ourselves in cotton wool and, as a result, our bodies have become lazy – but in reality, we have the capability to be far more physically and mentally resilient than we realise...

hormesis: the game-changer

Short and specific periods of controlled stress allows a dormant power to be tapped into and, amazingly, stimulates cellular changes within the body that can create extraordinary results. These multiple health benefits can include everything from increased energy levels, to better quality sleep, sharpened cognitive clarity, boosted immunity, balanced digestion and healthy weight loss. Most of all, brief, controlled stress has proven to have profound effects on longevity within the body. This process is called hormesis, which comes from the ancient Greek word for 'setting in motion,' and has been studied since the late nineteenth century.

Hormesis delivers a physical and mental reset that is equivalent to an entire upgrade for the body's systems and works by slightly damaging proteins, tissue and organisms. Cells react to the stressor, whether it be fasting over controlled periods of time, doing exercise or taking a freezing cold shower, and while it may not feel good initially, the body begins to acclimatise to what it is experiencing – and this is where the magic happens.

It responds to this short-lived stress by clearing up the damaged cells or stimulating their repair through a process called autophagy. It's like an evolution of sorts takes place with the body where it's adapting to the situation to emerge stronger and more resilient both biologically and emotionally. Yes – becoming a Marvel superhero is easier than you think.

the outrageous magic of autophagy

Human beings are basically walking, talking masses of cells. These cells form tissues, which form organs, which form us. Cells are highly skilled, but life is not easy for them. They spend their whole existence tirelessly working, until eventually they start to fall apart or fail and end up killing themselves. They are programmed to die through a process called apoptosis, which happens when the body perceives them as damaged beyond repair, but it often happens a bit prematurely – like taking a car to the crusher just because the handbrake stopped working.

Obviously we don't want inefficient cells dragging around the body not doing their jobs properly – but in some cases, these cells could be revived and rebooted if they just had their failing handbrakes replaced.

This is where autophagy comes in – a form of cell rehab triggered by hormesis that offers an alternative to certain death. Autophagy (from the ancient Greek 'auto', meaning 'self', and 'phagy', meaning 'eating') is a natural process which stimulates cell repair by 'eating' or removing the component part that is failing so the cell can renew itself and therefore prevent it from having to fall on its own sword.

Science has revealed that autophagy acts like a dramatic spring clean. It reduces the need for apoptosis and the energy this process requires to work by increasing failing cells' functionality and lifespan. It's a far more efficient recycling process where the beneficial results vastly outweigh the initial stress that the cells experience.

When damaged components within the cells are not cleared out through autophagy, the cells fail to divide and they use excess energy to keep themselves going, which clutters up the body – it's like not clearing the sweet wrappers out of your car. Not only does this drain the body, it is also very ageing and can lead to age-related disease.

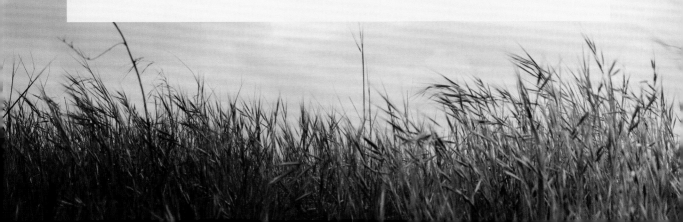

That is why it's common to feel a huge improvement in multiple ways after putting the body through autophagy. Coupled with hormesis, autophagy increases resilience and ultimately leads to the body feeling completely transformed.

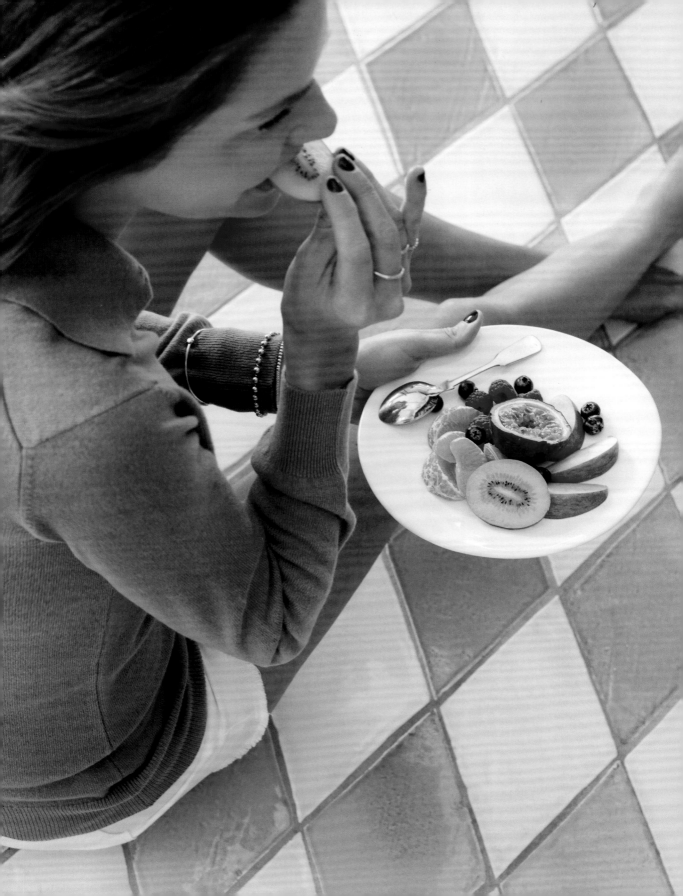

our bad marriage with food

Put your biscuits down and listen up. If you really want to turn autophagy up to 11, the best way is to temporarily deprive the body of nutrients through fasting. I understand that the concept of fasting may sound a bit (said in a tiny voice) terrifying, particularly in an age where so many of us in the West are surrounded by food. Walking down the street, we'll pass a supermarket, a café, a restaurant or a sandwich bar within minutes. A few clicks on an app and someone will deliver food to our door. Food is around every corner, ready and waiting to be eaten whenever we feel like it. Yum, yum, yum.

We're also not working the fields for our bread in the same way our ancestors did, and that created a disconnect. Our relationship with food can be mindless. It's part of what has made life too cosy – and there is scientific evidence to prove it.

Research has shown not only that Western diets are high in calories and low in nutrients, but also that we're over-eating. As a result, our bodies are not performing at the level they could and should be. Like putting the wrong petrol in a car, it means our systems simply cannot function in the way they are meant to.

Excess weight does not just come from a high calorie diet. It's also a reflection of nutrient deficiency. Without nutrients, the body cannot continually regulate an onslaught of calories – and this makes it impossible to maintain a healthy weight.

Before you throw this book across the room, screaming as you immediately order a Chinese takeaway, let me soothe your nerves by clarifying that fasting is not about starvation. It's about concentrated spells of calorie restriction. A reduction of as little as 10–15 per cent has been scientifically proven to significantly improve health and slow biological ageing, by switching on the body's longevity genes. Throw some time-restricted eating into the mix and you're really cooking with gas. (Except you're not cooking, you're starving – no, fasting. It's different.) We need only look to the Blue Zones and their cheerful, youthful centenarians having boozy dinners at midnight for evidence of this.

fasting explained in 30 seconds

FOOD RELEASES ENERGY!

Eating triggers the body to release glucose (sugar) into the bloodstream, which is picked up by the hormone insulin and distributed around the body to be used as energy. This supply can typically last for around three hours and is known as the anabolic or 'fed' state.

ACCESS THE EMERGENCY RESERVES!

When the glucose supply in the bloodstream has been exhausted, the body will turn to its energy reserves, which are stored as glycogen in the liver and muscles (known as the catabolic state). When these reserves are empty, the liver releases ketones (chemicals produced when the liver breaks down fat), which supply the body with energy during a process called ketosis. Autophagy now gets going.

The time it takes to move from a catabolic state to ketosis will vary from person to person depending on several factors – what they've eaten, how active they've been and how much energy they've used up, as well as lifestyle, genetics and general health. Having a good diet, eating in a time-restricted window and being active will allow the body to enter the state of ketosis much faster. Reach for your sprouting grains – and run!

it's getting hot/cold in here!
heat and cold exposure

There are, of course, many other ways beyond food to create hormetic stress. Exposing the body to extreme heat or cold is a wellness tradition that dates back thousands of years. Visiting the baths with their warm, hot and cold rooms was a daily ritual for ancient Romans of all classes. The Berber tradition of being buried in scorching hot desert sand to ease joint pain has seen a resurgence in recent years, while Nordic and Eastern European countries have long practised swimming in icy waters throughout winter. See? It's not just me making you do this stuff.

For centuries, humans have naturally gravitated to the restorative power of hot and cold exposure, blissfully unaware of the science behind it. There's a simple reason why – the effects feel fantastic. And that's because, in spite of being sweaty and red-faced or swearing through chattering teeth, amazing things are happening within the body.

When we are exposed to intense heat or cold, the body activates stress proteins – heat-shock proteins (HSP) and cold-shock proteins (CSP). The 'trauma' of these stressors triggers metabolic processes that quickly act to try and restore homeostasis – and with this comes huge benefits.

One of the most significant processes happens within the body's cells. Proteins are the main component of a cell and are essential to its health. They fulfil their role within a cell by going through a process called 'protein folding', but this doesn't always go smoothly. Proteins can fold incorrectly, potentially cluttering the cell and leaving it damaged or dead – and unhealthy cells like these can lead to the development of diseases or premature ageing.

During exposure to heat and cold, this cell stress response acts as a protective mechanism to help the body adapt to what is happening. HSP and CSP target cells containing badly folding proteins, intervene, and help them properly refold. They also support new proteins by ensuring they fold in the right way. Like the ultimate laundry service. This also helps you look and feel younger. Be still, my heart.

Heat exposure raises the heart rate and causes the body to sweat, similarly to exercising, as well as stimulating the lymphatic system to flush out toxins, which is always a winner. Cold exposure can even turn the body's white fat (the inactive storage kind we use to keep us cushioned and warm) to brown fat (the metabolic kind that burns energy like muscle does to help regulate our core temperature).

Brown fat, which is the layer that lives just under the skin, starts to reduce as we age. Not only can cold exposure help the body to develop more of it, but also it activates the mitochondria to help the body burn more energy. Increased levels of brown fat come with all kinds of health benefits, from balancing cholesterol and insulin levels to helping keep arteries and bones healthy. Brown fat is good. We love brown fat. Brown fat burns white fat. Brown fat wins.

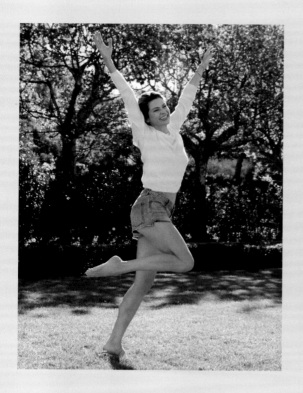
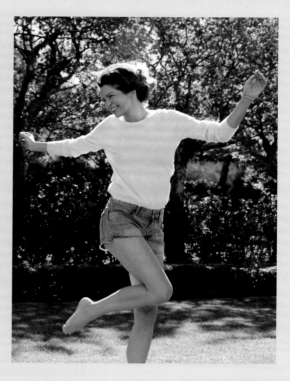
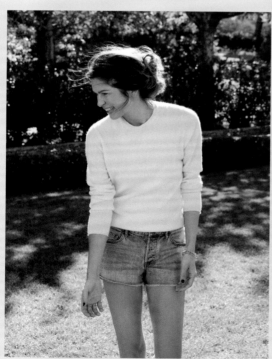
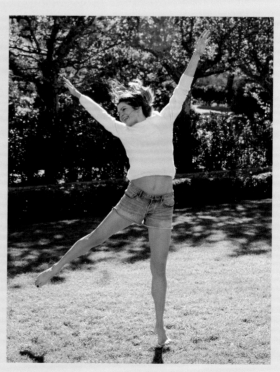

drop and give me ten!
exercise

We all know we should probably be doing more exercise – particularly as we've become a very sedentary bunch, sitting around all day staring at our computers. All exercise is beneficial, but particular types are specific to improving longevity – for example, the more strenuous, strengthening, sweaty, out-of-breath or resistance training kind. I know you're excited to read that. Muscle is an essential component of healthy ageing, but it needs to be stimulated through the stress of exercising in order to develop.

So there you are in the gym lifting weights or on the Pilates Reformer and you are screaming on the inside (and maybe just actually screaming). What exactly is going on? Exercising effectively damages muscle. It causes tiny tears (sounds terrifying, but it really isn't), which stimulates the growth-supporting protein enzyme mTOR and muscle stem cells, along with hormones like testosterone and insulin growth factor, to repair the area affected. This response fuses muscle fibres together, not just helping them to recover but building on what was there before.

This may come with initial muscle soreness, but it is an important part of the process that develops muscle and a greater tolerance for exercise, which improves fitness and strength. Each time this kind of hedonic adaptation raises the bar on what the body considers its baseline.

Exercise lessens the release of pro-inflammatory cytokines, which can cause systemic inflammation. This creates a healthier environment in which the body's systems are able to thrive. Regular physical activity is also key to reducing excess weight and the inflammation that comes with it. Exercise puts out fires left, right and centre.

Research has also shown that regular exercise assists the body in clearing itself of senescent cells – the redundant kind that drift about, getting in the way. The type of strengthening physical activity where you're out of breath (known as hypoxia) improves oxygen circulation and extends the lifespan of telomeres (the little caps on the end of a cell that diminish every time it divides, see page 16) and this supports the cells to live longer. Be cheered by all of this next time you stagger out of the gym, cursing your wobbling legs.

the more stressed your plants, the better *diet*

When it comes to food, autophagy is not just triggered by when you eat, but can be induced by what you eat. All thanks to a compound found in certain types of plant-based foods that mimic the ways in which fasting stresses the body – and it does this by stimulating SIRT longevity genes to release the sirtuin enzymes that trigger autophagy.

These sirtuin-activating compounds (STACs) can be found in polyphenols – plant chemicals that are known to significantly increase sirtuin activity. Some are more famous than others – resveratrol, for example, is found in red wine (casually drop that into conversation next time you open a bottle). Its lesser known companions include Indole-3-carbinol (I3C) found in cruciferous vegetables like broccoli, cauliflower and kale; and quercetin, found in onions, citrus fruit and green tea. So yes, as strange as it might sound, eating stressed plants is actually good for you.

plants get stressed?

Hang on, you're thinking. Plants get stressed? The answer is: yes. Plants have to navigate choppy waters just like the rest of us – okay, perhaps they don't have to worry about filing tax returns or getting divorced, but plant life is not without its challenges. As plants can't run away from stressful situations, they instead produce phytonutrients (plant stress chemicals called polyphenols) when facing a perceived danger. In turn, when we eat a stressed plant, these phytonutrients stimulate the body's cellular protective mechanisms, helping us to become stronger, healthier and more resilient against factors like UV exposure, harmful bacteria and pollutants – and ultimately improve longevity. This is known as xenohormesis.

Research suggests that eating foods (or 'sirtfoods' as they've been nicknamed) packed with sirtuin activators like polyphenols has a similar anti-ageing effect on the body as intermittent fasting and a low-calorie diet, as well as an influence on how fat metabolises and manages healthy weight loss. This is the kind of thing that gets me up in the morning, FYI.

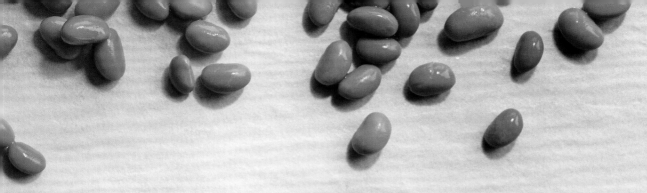

meet the sirtuins:
guardians of genomes

Forget *Guardians of the Galaxy*. As far as I'm concerned, the film that is begging to be made is Sirtuins: Guardians of the Genomes. Their mission is to nobly defend the body against premature ageing and illness by repairing DNA and preserving the genome's integrity. Come on, who wouldn't want to watch that?

This story starts with SIRT genes, which live within the body's cells mainly in the mitochondria or nucleus. Think of them as the body's crisis management team – a highly specialised emergency service that is activated in response to hormesis. When the siren sounds and the body experiences hormetic stress, SIRT genes trigger a response among the seven sirtuin enzymes (imaginatively named SIRT 1–SIRT 7), and these protective organisms are the biological catalysts for autophagy.

Experts in their field, the seven sirtuins work across organs and internal systems, and critically, one of these jobs is to reduce cellular senescence. They help to repair DNA that has become damaged through factors like oxidative stress, and they slow down the rate at which telomeres begin to shorten. Not only does this improve health and how the body feels in the here and now, but they are able to significantly influence healthy weight loss and slow down how the body ages. Clever.

It doesn't end there. Sirtuins not only produce mitochondria, they also improve its relationship with the cell nucleus so that it works more efficiently. They reduce inflammation and regulate insulin levels, decreasing the risk of age-related illnesses developing. By pausing normal activity to focus on survival, sirtuins work to restore homeostasis during hormetic stress. This protective mechanism helps the body to adapt to what it is experiencing by clearing out redundant cells, preserving energy, streamlining efficiency and increasing the speed at which chemical reactions take place. It is the ultimate in personal maintenance. If only we could employ sirtuins to do the school run or organise the house. Life would be so much easier.

What turns autophagy from a kitten to a lion is sirtuin activation, which is why they are considered the most important genes of all when it comes to longevity. Their influence on the ageing process is... how to put this? HUGE.

longevity and NAD+: a love story

NAD+ (officially named nicotinamide adenine dinucleotide, if you want to be formally introduced) is a coenzyme that lives within every living cell, speeding up chemical reactions within the body. Its job is to keep the cell's mitochondria healthy and functioning – put it this way, if the mitochondria is the cell battery, NAD+ is the battery charger. NAD+ molecules are energy generators for different systems all over the body – including sirtuins, which use them to regulate the metabolism and the circadian rhythm. They are essential for the immune system and keep our DNA healthy by protecting cells.

The bottom line is, NAD+ keeps us alive. It is so crucial, that without it, we would shrivel up like a vampire who forgot it was morning and went swanning out into the sun. Needless to say as we age, NAD+ levels begin to deplete because sirtuins need more and more of them and this reduction can contribute to age-related conditions. This is why they are key players in the long-game that is life. Fortunately, increased levels of NAD+ are a by-product of making longevity-supporting changes to diet and lifestyle and we'll be looking at how to initiate them later.

nutrient sensing pathways

This is the story of a power dynamic between four nutrient-sensing pathways: two of these, mTOR and IGF1, respond to nutrient levels, using them for all forms of growth in the body. The problem is, this anabolic reaction is great if you need to build muscle. However, it is less good for longevity, because the body needs to be in a catabolic state to experience autophagy.

Conversely, the other two pathways, sirtuins and AMPK, sense nutrient scarcity and hormetic stress (i.e. during fasting) and this makes them crucial for longevity. So while growth within the body is obviously important, it's also crucial that it doesn't run wild, but is instead regulated through intermittently pausing these processes through the autophagy cleansing process.

inflammation, immunity and longevity

And now we meet one of the big hitters when it comes to longevity and how the body ages: inflammation. We tend to think of inflammation as something bad, but most people live with gently fluctuating levels of it most of the time. Inflammation plays a critical role in how the immune system operates. We need it – but there are two types of inflammation and it's important to understand the differences between them.

acute inflammation – *the hero*

Acute inflammation is the emergency response to injury or illness. Inflammatory hormones stimulate blood flow to the damaged tissue, increasing the speed at which immune cells can be rushed to the scene and start their work in resolving the situation. This is why inflammation typically causes redness and swelling. The same is true of a blocked nose – inflammation causes the mucous membranes in the nasal passages to produce more fluid to help flush out the infection. It's like police tape is being put up around the problem before the ambulance arrives. As with most things, inflammation is at its most effective and balanced when we are young and everything is working like clockwork. Typical.

chronic inflammation – *the villain*

Chronic inflammation is significantly less helpful. It's the black sheep of the inflammation family. This occurs when inflammation doesn't go away after its job is done. In fact, it hangs around causing cell and tissue damage, it helps to develop diseases, builds fat and yes – contributes to the ageing process in an ex- tremely disruptive, 'nobody asked for your help' way. It can be hard to detect, but if left untreat- ed, can create havoc for years.

and then there's inflammaging…

The impact of chronic or constant low- grade inflammation on longevity is known as 'inflammaging'. It has a huge influence on how the body ages. Inflammaging is when pro-inflammatory cytokines (a kind of messenger protein produced by immune cells) begin to outnumber anti-inflammatory cytokines, throwing off the immune system's response, which leaves the body with excessive inflammation. This can disrupt the body's ability to get back to normal and ultimately can cause damage to soft tissue and glands.

Intestinal microbiome imbalance, immune cell senescence and high levels of cell debris are all fellow contributors to inflammaging – but the big one is excess weight. Carrying too much body fat will stimulate chronic inflammation in the body. Then the flood gates open to all kinds of potential health conditions. This is what makes inflammaging so important to manage. It can sit around in the background like a silent assassin, narrowing arteries, mutating cells and causing blood pressure to spike – none of which will leave anyone feeling good. Quite the opposite.

Happily, inflammaging is not a given, as inflammation is in constant fluctuation. The way we live our lives has a huge impact on its ever changing levels. While stress, lack of sleep, high-sugar diets, nutritional deficiencies and not enough exercise can all start to wear the body down over the years, they are also within our control to change.

why weight matters to longevity

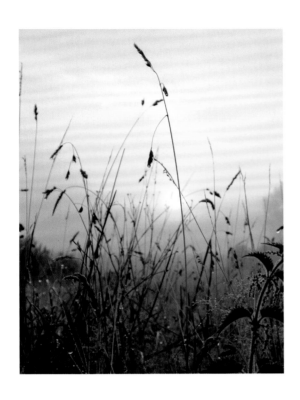

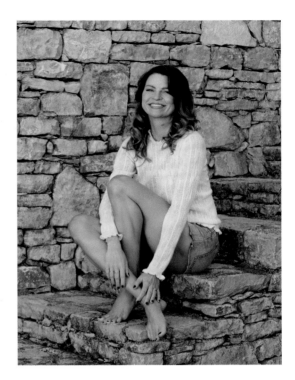

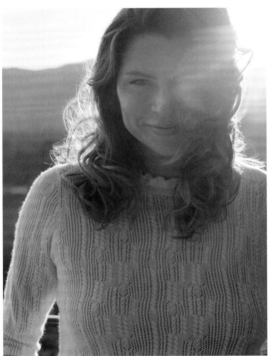

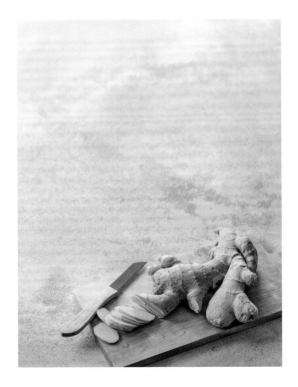

why weight matters…

We all know the importance of being a healthy weight – but it's particularly interesting to look at in the context of how our body ages. We now understand that too much fat increases inflammaging and that, in turn, amplifies the body's ageing process. Being a healthy weight is so crucial, I feel like I should get in a plane and write it across the sky:

'PLEASE BE A HEALTHY WEIGHT. APART FROM ALL THE OTHER GOOD THINGS ABOUT IT, YOU WILL AGE BETTER.'

That kind of thing.

So let's talk about weight loss. It's easy to imagine it involves simply getting rid of as much fat as possible, but there's far more to it than that. We actually need fat. It protects, insulates and stores energy. However, we constantly walk a tightrope with our fat. Too little fat and you're in trouble. Too much fat and you're also in trouble. Somewhere in the middle and you're cooking with gas. As with most things in life, it's all about balance.

Our relationship with our body fat tends to reflect our desire to look good – which is nothing to be ashamed of – but we also need to be aware of how unmanaged, excess fat can cause damage to our health both now and in the long term. This is why we should start to think of weight loss as not just about being slimmer, but, more importantly, about being healthy, stronger and fitter.

Being overweight can reduce life expectancy by several years. That's a pretty startling thought. Having too much unnecessary fat may lead to insulin resistance, heart problems, cognitive conditions and chronic inflammation, as well as metabolic and hormonal disruption. And that's before we've even got to how it influences the ageing process. Here's the long and short of it: maintaining a healthy weight throughout your life is one of the most significant investments you can make for yourself now and as you continue to age over the years.

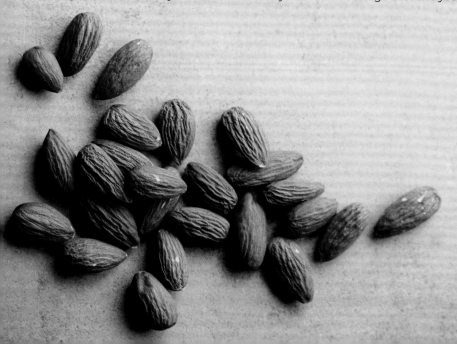

fat. the facts.

Fat comes in two forms. The unpopular white kind, which stores energy and we're always trying to get rid of because it makes our favourite jeans too tight; and the heroic brown, metabolic kind, which generates heat, keeps us warm and burns calories. Both kinds also cushion and protect us. We need the stuff. It is critical to our survival.

ghrelin and leptin

The stomach lining secretes the hunger hormone ghrelin, which stimulates appetite. Its levels peak in anticipation of eating.

Known as the satiety hormone, leptin is secreted from mainly fat cells. Its job is to manage appetite and energy levels; it tells the hypothalamus when the body has had enough to eat.

Too much leptin can actually desensitise the brain's response to it. Instead of feeling satisfied, the brain tricks the body into thinking it's still hungry and needs to eat more. It thinks it needs to store more fat – which it doesn't – and this is known as leptin resistance.

how does fat form in the first place?

When food is eaten, glucose enters the bloodstream. The body releases insulin from the pancreas to collect the glucose and transport it to the mitochondria within the cells for energy production. Insulin helps to regulate, convert and activate glucose. Important job.

The body needs a certain amount of glucose for immediate use because it needs to maintain ever-fluctuating levels of energy. However, anything it doesn't need straight away gets transformed into glycogen and stored in the liver and muscles. When those storage spaces are full, excess glycogen is transformed again into triglycerides, a type of fat, and stored in adipose tissue. Unlike liver and muscle cells, adipose tissue doesn't have a limit on how much it can store. You can see where we're going with this.

A diet that is high in carbohydrates or sugar makes the pancreas keep having to produce insulin to cope with the influx of glucose in its efforts to stabilise blood sugar levels. This makes the body think it has plenty of energy available for immediate use and therefore need not turn to its stored reserves in adipose tissue. In fact, what it believes instead is that it should be storing more. Hello, weight gain.

excess weight and inflammation
– the gruesome twosome

Once upon a time, excess weight asked inflammation out on a date. They got on like a house on fire and became the couple nobody wanted to know and were never invited anywhere.

Why is this grim pairing such a problem? Gaining weight triggers inflammation, but, curiously, as a kind of innate immune response. It seems excess levels of fat cells are perceived as an injury or infection, so the body responds by sending along pro-inflammatory cytokines and immune cells to where excess fat has collected.

If the problem were actually an injury or infection, this emergency response would be temporary. Unfortunately, excess adipose tissue that is not dealt with continues to over-stimulate the immune system. This is when inflammation can become chronic, disrupting the balance of the body's metabolism.

This results in adipose tissue itself becoming very inflammatory, spreading more inflammation to its neighbouring organs and tissue like a wildfire, which in turn contributes to systemic inflammation within the body as a whole; this is a classic hallmark of ageing. Think of the longest lines of dominoes possible, but on fire.

Weight gain is a vicious circle. The more inflammation you have, the more prone you become to gaining weight. That's why being overweight can be described as a form of 'low-grade chronic inflammation' with the potential to lead to insulin resistance and type 2 diabetes, making it harder to lose weight, but easier to keep gaining it. Arrgh!

Excess weight can damage your body, your health and the way you're ageing. It sounds dramatic, but honestly, it can determine the course of your life – even how long you'll live. Before you start packing your bags to move to the moon because this is all getting a bit scary, let's circle back to the power you have over your weight. It's a lot. And every change you implement, no matter how small, is a step in the right direction to restoring balance and changing the future of your health.

how does body composition fit into this?

It's impossible to talk about weight loss without including body composition. Let's think about scales for a moment. In reality, they are extremely misleading and only tell part of the story. The body is composed of muscle, organs, bone, tissue and fluids, as well as fat – so the idea that you'd stand on a set of scales and cast judgement on how 'fat' you think you are really doesn't make sense, as it doesn't take into account all the other components of your body the scales are weighing.

Muscle is heavier than fat – that's why exercising more may make the scales go up instead of down. It is also metabolically active, meaning it needs to burn glucose to create energy in order to help the body move. In stark contrast, fat doesn't need energy to function, so healthy weight loss needs to strike the right balance between muscle mass and necessary fat. Scales make it hard for us to see the whole picture, and that can be damaging. Are we really going to judge our own self-worth by a number on a device? No thanks.

Muscle also plays a protective role by producing chemicals that reduce inflammation, all of which contribute to rebalancing the negative effects of ageing. As we age, we typically become less active. That's why we tend to gain fat and lose muscle mass. Body composition can shift without us even realising – we may look the same, but inside, fat will start to replace muscle mass. By the age of 30, muscle mass typically starts to decline, but this can be completely turned around by regular exercise.

Healthy muscle mass actually signals bones to keep themselves strong. Having an active lifestyle increases quality of life in so many ways, so you need to use it before you lose it. Put simply, while it's completely normal to experience a decrease in muscle mass as we age, you can rebalance it with dietary and lifestyle interventions. Balanced muscle mass and body composition are the key to health and longevity. If we take care of both, we change everything.

how do I know if I'm a healthy weight?

Most of us are aware if we start to put on a kilo or so just from how our clothes fit. If you want to take a closer look at what might be happening with your weight, body composition scales will give a far more accurate reading than regular scales, as they'll take into account the weight of your muscle mass and other components.

You can also do some calculations yourself, such as BMI, which measures height and weight ratios, but it's worth bearing in mind that these calculations give a far more general picture. The Waist to Hip ratio (WHR) is popular in the medical community and is often used in conjunction with BMI calculation, but, really, you'll know in yourself if things are changing rather than depending on a number system to tell you. Also they're really complicated maths equations, and wouldn't you rather just be having a nice drink or going for a longevity-supporting run around the park than fiddling around with difficult sums?

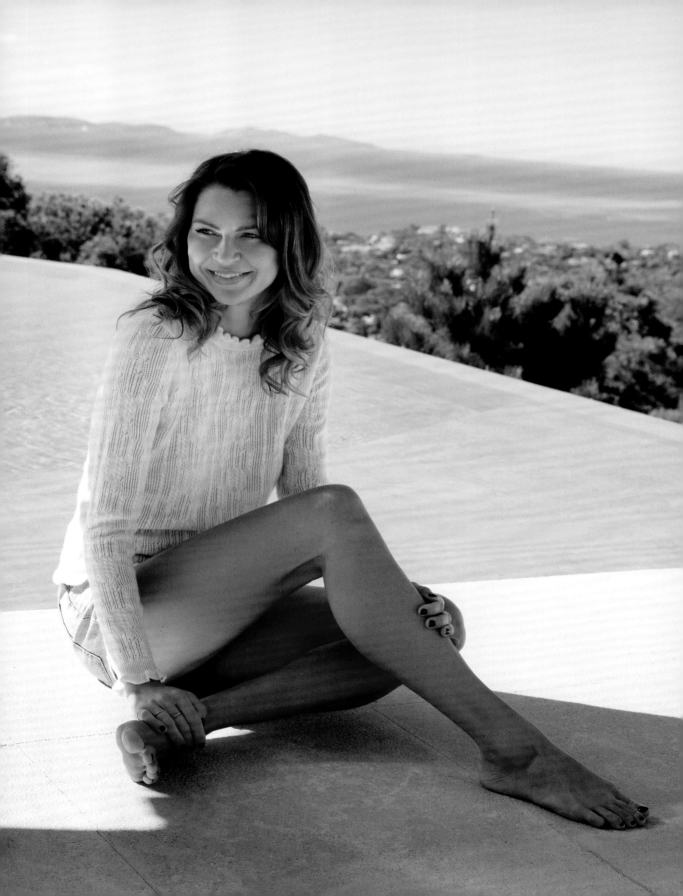

what are calories?

Calories are found in food and drink and are little units of energy that take the form of heat. The body cannot function without energy and uses calories to either generate or store it. In a straightforward world, 100 calories of kale and 100 calories of cinnamon roll would produce the same amount of energy. But there's a small thing called nutritional value that makes it all a bit complicated. Full of nutrients, antioxidants and fibre, kale delivers a power-packed punch of goodness to the body, burning energy to be digested. Cinnamon rolls with their simple carbohydrates and sugar, send blood sugar levels skyrocketing and then crashing, while also needing almost no energy to be digested. Too much of one and not enough of the other can lead to weight gain. See if you can work out which.

metabolism and basal metabolic rate:
what's going on with these two?

Metabolism is an essential chemical process that combines the calories in everything the body eats and drinks with oxygen and converts them into energy.

The basal metabolic rate (BMR) refers to the baseline number of calories the body needs in its resting state – because regardless of whether we're sitting still, reading or even sleeping, our body still needs energy to help us breathe, balance our hormone levels, digest, repair cells, grow, think, pump our blood – to keep us, well, alive.

Lots of factors will determine how someone's BMR is calculated. Men tend to have more muscle, less fat and burn more calories than women of the same age and weight. Muscle mass typically decreases with age, while fat levels may increase, resulting in fewer calories being burnt. And then there's body composition. Those who have more muscle or are just physically larger specimens burn more calories.

If your BMR is calculated to be 1,000 calories a day, that means your body will burn 1,000 calories a day in a resting state. This number remains pretty consistent throughout life.

However, beyond BMR, other factors use up calories, of course. Thermogenesis is the process by which the body burns energy to regulate its temperature. 3–10 per cent of calorie intake is burned through digestion. And then there's physical activity – everything from the deliberate kind like walking to a destination, exercise or sport to the non-deliberate kind, like moving around the house or even just fidgeting. The body needs energy for all of it. Therefore, it's possible to eat more calories than the number identified in a BMR calculation as long as they are used for other purposes.

how blood sugar affects weight and metabolism

The process of digestion releases glucose from food that has been eaten, but the rate at which it travels into the bloodstream and how it behaves when it gets there depends on three things – what was eaten, when it was eaten and how it was eaten. Will the release of glucose be gentle and steady through the course of the day or will it be lurching all over the place, peaking and falling?

Blood sugar levels impact everything from appetite, sleep and cravings, to even mental health. Keeping them balanced is so key to how you will feel in so many areas of life that it's not even funny. Put it this way – if you're distracted reading this because you'd rather be eating a packet of chocolate biscuits, chances are your blood sugar levels could do with a serious talking to.

► WHAT ARE YOU EATING?

Here's a clue – simple carbohydrates will spike blood sugar levels because they're low on nutrients and fibre and are more likely to be stored as excess fat.

Complex carbohydrates have a considerably higher fibre content, which means they get broken down and released into the bloodstream much more slowly.

Now we're talking.

► WHEN ARE YOU EATING?

Waiting until you feel hungry rather than just peckish means blood sugar levels have taken a nose-dive. It's much better to get in there first with regular healthy snacks between meals.

► HOW ARE YOU EATING?

The best way to ensure a slow, steady release of sugars into the bloodstream is to always have a balance – that means protein, complex carbohydrates and healthy fats with every meal or snack.

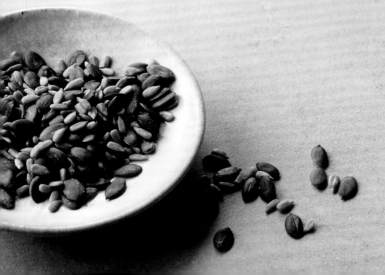

unsustainable weight loss plans

Finding the right weight loss plan can be a challenge. For any chance of success, it needs to be realistic in terms of what it's demanding of you. Otherwise, the experience is just deeply stressful and won't have any lasting impact beyond the inevitable initial weight loss. This is why most crash diets don't work in the long term and the weight that may have been lost tends to make a pretty rapid return after the diet has ended. The plan needs to fit into the reality of everyday life and change eating habits for the better – that means when the odd fluctuation happens, which is perfectly normal, it becomes easier and easier to drop a kilo whenever needed. It simply requires making small adjustments to a greatly improved overall diet rather than a huge overhaul. And this is the key to keeping the weight off.

healthy weight doesn't exist in isolation

The human body is intricately interconnected and any disruption has a knock-on effect. Poor sleep can lead to an inability to lose weight. Blood sugar levels affect energy and stress, impacting immunity and hormones. If internal systems are imbalanced, the body prioritises restoring equilibrium before turning its attention to weight loss.

stress, sleep and weight gain

Believe it or not, stress plays a huge role in weight gain. A constant stream of the stress hormone cortisol can increase appetite and spike blood sugar levels. This can make the body resistant to insulin, causing havoc with sleep and creating an imbalance of hormones like leptin and ghrelin (the pair that regulate the appetite), which are typically metabolised at night. Without this night time housekeeping, many of the body's systems face an uphill struggle to function at a normal level. When the body feels tired, it often craves sugar, which obviously leads to weight gain. And being quite grumpy.

intestinal microbiota

Microbiota – otherwise known as the trillions of bacteria that live in the digestive tract – play an enormous role in the body's health. And not just on how efficiently nutrients are absorbed, processed and transported. The state of our microbiota also influences the immune system, energy levels, appetite and cognitive and mental health. An imbalanced microbiota has not only been shown to impair the ability to lose weight, but also can lead to intestinal inflammation and then systemic inflammation and inflammaging. All the inflammations, all of the time. Do not underestimate the power of a happy, healthy microbiota, not only in day-to-day health but also in how the body will age.

5

the transformative power of intermittent fasting

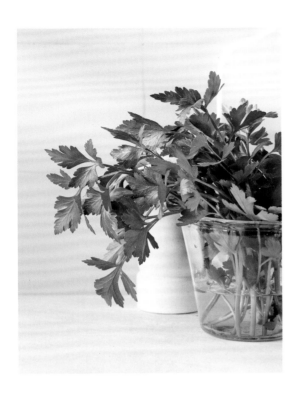
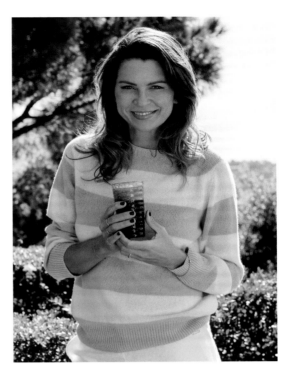
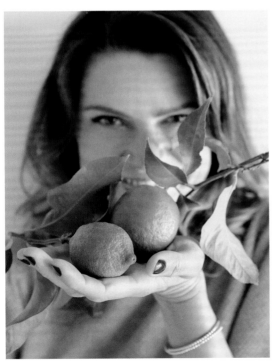
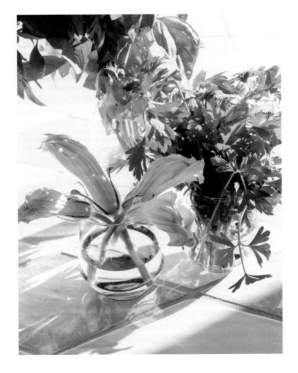

what is intermittent fasting?

Intermittent fasting (IF) involves controlled periods of eating and fasting and is the umbrella term for many of today's most popular weight loss plans (time-restricted eating, calorie-restricted diets, 5:2 and alternate-day fasting). It is the most researched and impactful form of weight loss, with scientific evidence to prove the numerous beneficial effects it has on general health and longevity.

In all my years as a nutritionist, the profound physical and mental changes that I've seen IF produce in my clients in such a short period of time never fails to amaze me. What IF does for the body is truly transformative. I love it not only because its foundations are in science, but also because it's sustainable. IF programmes are simple to follow and, crucially, they fit into the rhythm of everyday life without major disruption and that's what makes them so easy to return to whenever needed. Using IF as a foundation, I have now developed new longevity plans that turbo-charge the natural autophagy element that occurs with IF, revolutionising how the body ages.

I think of these as more than just longevity weight loss plans – they are a way of life where new habits are created and better choices become easier and easier to make. IF enables people to take control of their general health, mental health, weight, sleep, energy levels and more with minimal disruption. It really has the power to change the course of your life.

It's worth remembering that we are all biochemically different and may well have different goals, which is why I consider a one-plan-fits-all approach to be unrealistic. Some may want to achieve weight loss, some may want to boost autophagy and some may want to focus on rebalancing and improving sleep or energy levels. IF does it all – and my ethos is that there is a plan that works for everyone based on individual needs.

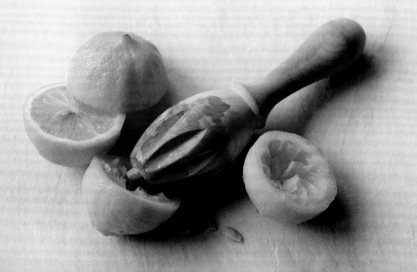

why not just restrict calories all the time?

Long term calorie restriction leads to an initial drop in weight, but will ultimately result in what is known as metabolic adaptation. This is when the body starts to panic about when its next refuel will happen and, as a result, stores energy in fat cells as an emergency back-up. This slowing down of the metabolism when calorie restriction is enforced over long periods of time means that the body is adapting to what is happening and any positive effects will radically slow down. Without entering a proper fasting state, the beneficial side effects reduce – ketone production will be lower because the body is still receiving glucose and autophagy isn't triggered to its full capacity. In contrast, IF keeps the body on its toes with temporary calorie restriction balanced with time-restricted eating. This means the body won't panic, but will instead lose weight healthily while also triggering autophagy.

what are the benefits of IF?

1 say goodbye to visceral fat

IF works in two ways when it comes to weight loss. One is the controlled reduction of calorie intake, which ideally means consuming less, putting the body into a calorie deficit. The second is it triggers ketosis and autophagy. This enhances and rebalances several crucial hormone functions to break down fat cells, including lowering insulin levels and increasing the metabolic rate. More calories are used than consumed, which drives weight loss.

IF targets visceral fat, the mean inflammatory kind that collects around the abdomen that can cause serious health problems. It preserves muscle mass, which is often one of the first things that takes a hit with less healthy diets, maintaining a balanced body composition. Next thing we know, it'll help us predict Grand National winners or lottery numbers – that's how clever it is. Science will discover this soon.

2 less inflammation

Autophagy has a radical effect on how the immune system actually produces its cells and even on their quality. Reducing nutrient intake during fasting drives the body to clear out or repair compromised immune cells. This also stimulates the production of new, fighting fit cells, upgrading the immune response in its entirety to function at a far higher level.

One of the major benefits of this is the effect it has on chronic inflammation – the dreaded companion of excess weight and ageing. Studies have shown that fasting reduces the number of monocytes (which secrete pro-inflammatory cytokines) moving around the body. These pro-inflammatory cells duck and dive around in the bloodstream and have the potential to cause severe damage to tissues and organs – a problem that has become prevalent for many people in recent years because of bad eating habits. Periods of fasting actually put monocytes into 'sleep mode' and even makes them less inflammatory.

3 better immunity

Fasting has also been shown to improve the memory of immune cells, which is a central component of how they work. During an illness or infection, immune cells learn to recognise invading pathogens. If they turn up again, the immune system will remember how to deal with them. Autophagy is able to improve their memories. Like microscopic elephants, they forget nothing.

4 sleep at night

It's easy to imagine that an IF plan might make you feel more tired than normal, as the body seems to be doing so much work beneath the surface. In fact, energy levels go up. One of the reasons for this is the effect IF has on sleep. Scientific research has shown that within just a week of intermittent fasting, sleep is vastly improved. Everything – from waking up in the night, being unable to settle, thrashing around and getting twitchy limbs – settles down and allows the body to sleep properly.

Another interesting point to note is that IF means eating less, which has a direct link to better sleep. Going to bed on a stomach that is not full will help the brain synchronise itself with the digestive system and circadian rhythm so that everything is working towards the same goal – shutting down for the night.

IF also stimulates a rise in melatonin, the sleep-inducing hormone, allowing for a significantly better quality and more restful night's sleep, as well as boosting human growth hormones (HGH) responsible for

general housekeeping and the cell repair that happens overnight.

5 bounce all day

Better sleep means increased energy during the day, with a bonus side order of improved concentration and stabilised moods.

Mitochondria, the energy hubs of the cell Mitochondria, the energy hubs of the cell, are specifically targeted during this mild form of stress (mitohormesis), triggering a protective response that increases their resilience. Alongside this, the energy used by dwindling cells to keep themselves going is also freed up, thanks to autophagy, which either clears them up or repairs them. This all ultimately leads to greater energy levels, better cellular function and healthy longevity.

6 a sharper, well-fed brain

The brain loves ketones. In the absence of glucose during fasting, the liver burns adipose tissue as fuel and this is when ketones are produced – a superfood for the brain. They have the unusual ability to cross the blood–brain barrier and fire the brain up so that mental clarity is noticeably sharper. Ketones are extremely valuable for those experiencing neurodegenerative conditions and other diseases associated with ageing. Put simply, fasting is like taking your brain on a deluxe spa weekend.

7 a hearty heart

IF improves heart health. It balances blood sugar levels, blood pressure, insulin production and cholesterol, and improves the symptoms of metabolic syndrome. This common condition causes symptoms including high blood pressure, insulin resistance, visceral fat and high levels of triglycerides, all of which can lead to a greater risk of heart-related health issues.

In its capacity to reduce chronic inflammation, IF also lowers the risk of blood vessels being damaged, which can often lead to heart conditions. And it's not all about avoiding problems – the heart improves functionality thanks to IF. It affects the way the body metabolises glucose and reduces 'bad' cholesterol (low-density lipoproteins, otherwise known as LDL), all of which impact body weight and the potential to develop diabetes. Quite understandably, the heart hearts IF.

8 a calm digestion and happy microbiome

THERE'S MORE. IF improves the function of the digestive system – of course it does. It allows the digestive tract to break from normal activity by temporarily not adding more to its workload. It allows it to focus on repairing issues that need addressing, calming down any adverse food reactions and eliminating waste matter from the digestive tract. It also amplifies fermentation and diversity of the microbiome, increasing its number of bacterial species and even the fatty acids that feed the beneficial bacteria. This is good news for digestion, but also for the immune system, as around 70 per cent of it resides in the digestive tract.

all roads lead to… longevity

It's not hard to see that cumulatively, all these extraordinary changes that take place during periods of IF will improve your health not only now, but also in the long term. Weight is balanced with muscle mass, the immune system is boosted and chronic inflammation is reduced. Good sleep helps to restore the body overnight and mitohormesis increases energy levels. Mental clarity and brain function are sharpened thanks to the influx of ketones. The cardiovascular system becomes more robust, as does the digestive system and microbiome.

This is a profound upgrade of cellular activity and it's all thanks to the spectacular transformative power of hormesis and autophagy. You might as well start planning your 200th birthday, because you'll probably still be here.

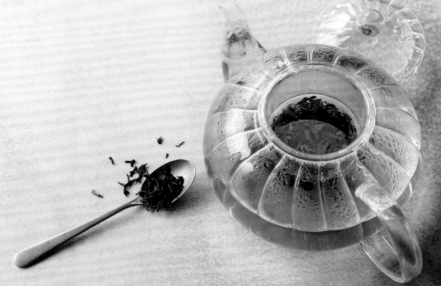

so what should I do?

Here's where things get really juicy. This is where you'll find out all the ways in which you can completely redirect how your body ages. From my longevity -stimulating intermittent fasting plans, advice on nutrition and lifestyle to physical activity and emotional wellbeing – with plenty of GP tips throughout. It only gets better from here...

6

the GP principles for a longevity diet

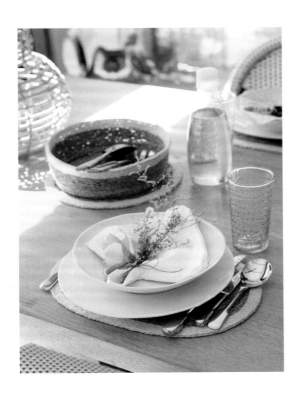
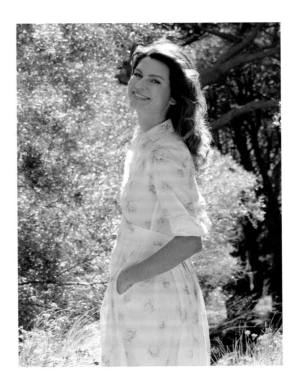
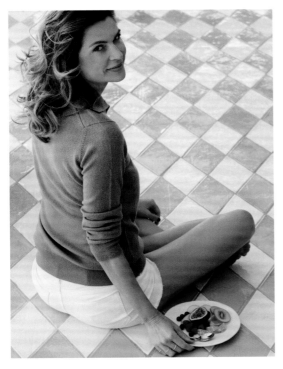
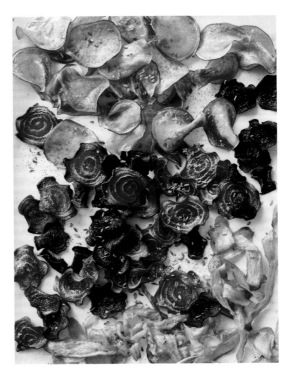

Before choosing which GP fasting plan you'd like to follow (see pages 82–95), it's important to understand some of my key nutrition principles and how they will serve you throughout the plans and beyond. The fasting plans are designed to reset the body, but beyond that, applying the right nutritional balance to everyday will ensure the best results.

Understanding how nutrition works and what the basic rules are will completely transform your body's biochemistry, affecting every internal system – from sleep, to energy levels, to mental clarity and immunity. As we've seen in the Blue Zones, the anti-ageing effects of certain diets are extraordinarily powerful and capable of radically changing lives for the better. It's no surprise that two out of the five Blue Zones are based on the Mediterranean diet in all its low-animal-protein, low-glycaemic-index and high-polyphenol deliciousness (while being drenched in olive oil and washed down with a glass of red).

My plans very rarely exclude food groups (unless it's medically necessary) – in fact, the opposite. Balance, as always, lies at the heart of everything – and opens the doors to a rich, varied world of healthy and nutritious food that will change the texture of everyday life.

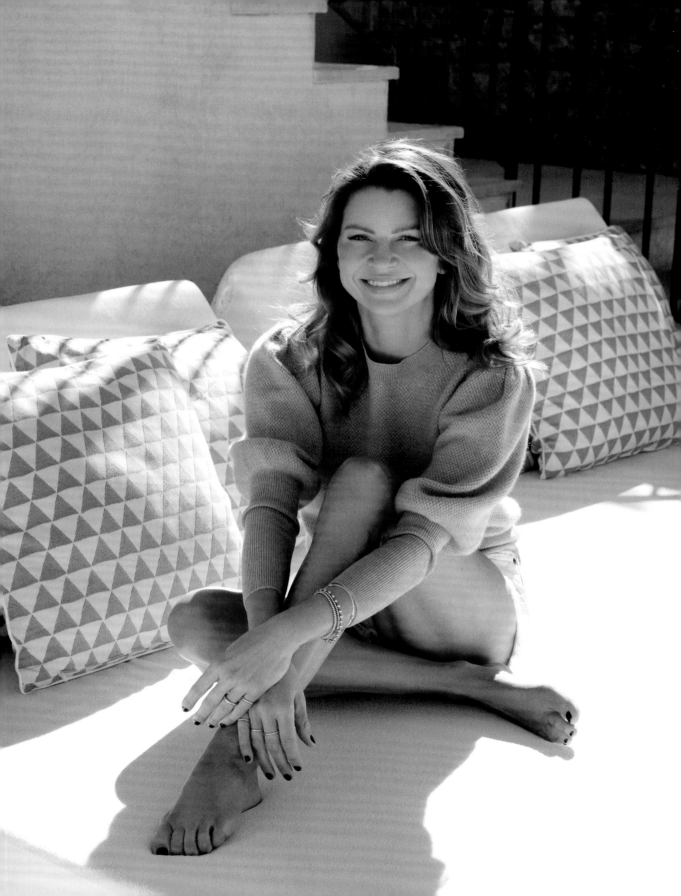

protein is everything

Protein is made of 20 amino acids, which carry out lots of important jobs in the body. They support muscle growth and lean muscle mass; balance blood sugar and insulin levels; manage the production of hormones and neurotransmitters; and repair cells as well as making new ones. It's easy to see that proteins are kind of a big deal. As the body produces only 11 of the 20 amino acids needed, the remaining 9 must come from what we eat.

Ditch starchy, sugary, nutrient-stripped white rice and replace it with high protein, longevity-loving super-grain quinoa.

animal vs plant: *the big question*

Protein plays an essential role in longevity, and variety is key to maximising its impact. It comes in two forms – animal and plant protein.

Animal protein is a complete protein and it contains all the amino acids we need from our diets, and is therefore a rich source. It also contains high levels of methionine and branched-chain amino acids, both of which are known to stimulate mTOR (the enzyme that regulates cell growth), the enemy of longevity. It's also known to aggravate inflammation. Naughty. As usual, there are no hard-and-fast rules about animal protein, so it's not a question of cutting it out entirely if you love it. It's about making it work for you. The best way to do this is to include plenty of fish, which is anti-inflammatory and packed with essential fatty acids, both of which support healthy longevity.

Plants are also fantastic protein sources, as they don't spike mTOR in the same way and contain beneficial fibre, vitamins, minerals and polyphenols (our friendly stress chemicals). Notably, Blue Zones have very high plant-protein diets, so there is empirical evidence that they help people live longer, healthier lives.

Think of red meat as a treat. Choose fresh (preferably organic), lean red meat over the cured or smoked varieties like salami, which are processed and full of chemicals.

Fish skin is sky-high in anti-inflammatory fatty acids, so don't discard it. Crisp it up in the oven or a frying pan and crunch it down with salt and olive oil. YUM.

plant proteins for the win

There's a huge variety of beneficial plant proteins. It's so good that even the incomplete kind, when combined, can provide the full profile of essential amino acids. Fermented plant-based products, such as miso, tofu and tempeh, are particularly good as they contain live bacteria, which makes them not only easily digestible, but extremely good for a thriving intestinal microflora.

Complete plant proteins:
► *quinoa, buckwheat, hemp seeds and chia seeds, blue-green algae (spirulina, chlorella and kelp), soya (edamame, tofu, tempeh, miso)*

Incomplete plant proteins:
► *wholegrains (rye, spelt, wheat, millet, oats), pulses (beans, chickpeas, lentils, peas), mushrooms, seeds, nuts, vegetables (spinach, broccoli, Brussels sprouts)*

Easy combinations:
► *Beans or lentils with nuts or seeds (lentils/chickpeas with pumpkin/sunflower seeds)*

► *Nuts or seeds with wholegrains (nut butter on rye or pumpernickel bread)*

► *Wholegrains with beans (beans and brown rice, hummus and oatcakes, bean dip with crackers)*

Algae is a nutritional super-bomb. Protein, polyphenols, minerals, antioxidants – you name it. It can come in powder form, so try adding a spoonful here and there to soups and smoothies for a revitalising mega-hit.

Earthy and delicious, mushrooms contain protein, are low in calories and are great for immunity. Try different varieties on toast or as a side dish, particularly the medicinal kind, such as shiitake, maitake, reishi, Cordyceps and lion's mane.

Maximise your plant-protein intake with vegan protein powders. The unflavoured kind can be added to pretty much anything, like soups, veggie stews, breakfast yogurt pots or cereal.

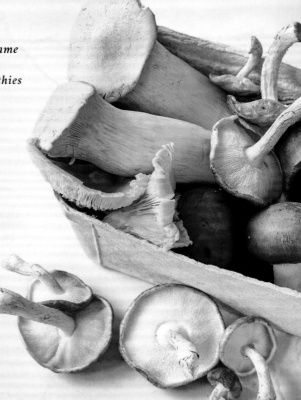

a note on nuts and seeds

Welcome to the easiest, healthiest, most convenient snack of them all: nuts and seeds. Eat them raw, flavoured, soaked overnight, in salads, in smoothies... anything, everything, all the time. Packing a protein punch, nuts and seeds are a rich source of vitamins, minerals, fibre and good fats.

▸ **Nuts:** *almonds, peanuts, Brazil nuts, macadamia nuts, hazelnuts, walnuts, cashew nuts*
▸ **Seeds:** *pumpkin, sunflower, chia, hemp, flax, sesame*

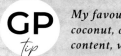

a little note on dairy

Fermented dairy products are far gentler on digestion because the fermentation process has effectively pre-digested the product before consumption. It also contains beneficial bacteria that are great for maintaining a robust intestinal microbiota and general health.

GP *tip*

My favourite longevity-loving dairy-free milks are nut (almond, cashew nut, hazelnut), coconut, oat, rice, soya and hemp. Choose unsweetened milks with a high protein content, which will be listed on the label.

GP *tip*

Hurray for dairy-free alternatives, which are widely available. We're talking soft cheeses, mozzarella and halloumi made from plant sources. Even some chocolate hazelnut spreads, yum, yum, yum.

GP *tip*

Flavoured vegan protein powders are great for people with a sweet tooth (kids love them too). Just mix with nut milk for a quick, healthy snack or add to a blender with some nuts, seeds, fruit and avocado.

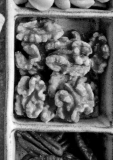

the complex world of carbohydrates

Vegetables, fruit, grains, pulses, nuts and seeds are all forms of carbohydrate, which are made of sugars, starches and fibres. Carbohydrates are a major source of energy for the body, which during digestion breaks them down into glucose that can be used immediately or stored for later.

Not all carbohydrates are created equal, as some have a higher sugar and fibre content than others. The glycaemic index (GI) rates carbohydrates eaten on their own from 0 to 100 (anything below 55 is considered low), but it's more helpful to look at total composition, taking into consideration the carbohydrate, fat and fibre content, how it's prepared, the serving size – and how all of these factors impact the release of glucose into the bloodstream. This measurement is known as the glycaemic load (GL) and gives a more accurate overall picture of how food affects blood sugar levels in real terms.

If sugary carbohydrates become too dominant in the diet, weight gain is just one of the side effects. It can actually accelerate the ageing process by continuously stimulating mTOR, raising inflammation levels, unbalancing hormones and increasing insulin resistance among its crimes. However, it's important to remember that the scale is an indication only; higher GI foods' number will reduce when eaten with proteins and fats – like pasta if it's served with Bolognese. Especially if the pasta is the wholegrain kind. Step forward to receive your medal.

another little note on sugar

Let's separate carbohydrates and sugars for a moment. Refined sugar is the mortal enemy of longevity; over-consumption of sugar is one of the primary causes of chronic inflammation and its merry band of diseases. Sugar stimulates the liver to produce fatty acids, and as the body tries to digest them, they release compounds that trigger the inflammatory process. The more sugar you eat, the worse it gets.

Don't be fooled by the promise of 'zero calories'. The taste of artificial sweeteners has been shown to still trigger the release of insulin, as happens with normal sugar, causing blood sugar imbalance, cravings and even weight gain. Yikes.

The sugar index is a minefield of multiple options. My preferred low GI sugars are agave syrup, xylitol, stevia and inulin. They all taste slightly different but are better options than refined sugar.

fibre – *what's the big deal?*

Fibre is a form of carbohydrate that the body cannot break down and is found in plant-based foods. It comes in two forms – soluble and insoluble. Fibre is incredibly important for maintaining healthy digestion because it helps clear out anything unusable as it passes through the body.

Insoluble fibre:	**Soluble fibre:**
Found in the outer coating or skin of vegetables and whole grains, it helps to keep digested food moving through the intestine.	Attracts water, which enables the body to pick up and clear out more redundant matter for excretion.
▶ **Insoluble fibre:** *fruit (raspberries, pears, apples, strawberries, oranges, bananas, pomegranates), vegetables (peas, broccoli, Brussels sprouts, cauliflower), nuts, seeds, lentils, beans, wholegrains (brown rice, buckwheat, quinoa, oats, barley)*	▶ **Soluble fibre:** *oats, barley, nuts (almonds, cashew nuts, hazelnuts, walnuts), seeds (flax, sunflower, pumpkin, hemp, chia), beans, lentils, peas, fruit (blueberries, blackberries, pears, raspberries, avocados, strawberries, kiwis, plums, figs, apricots), vegetables (spinach, sweet potatoes, broccoli, carrots)*

victorious vegetables

Vegetables are the kings of carbohydrates. What makes them especially beneficial is that not only are they rich in vitamins and minerals, but also they tend to be high in fibre and low in sugar, giving them a low GL. Vegetables come in two types – starchy and non-starchy. The starchy kind are higher in calories, so a portion of starchy potatoes would contain more calories than the same portion of non-starchy broccoli. This is one of the many reasons why non-starchy vegetables are excellent for weight management and longevity.

▶ **Starchy vegetables:** *potatoes, sweet potatoes, corn, parsnips, beans, peas, butternut squash, chickpeas, lentils*

▶ **Non-starchy vegetables:** *broccoli, kale, cauliflower, cabbage, asparagus, bean sprouts, Swiss chard, bok choy, Brussels sprouts, artichokes, aubergines, cucumber, spinach, courgettes*

GP *Tip*

If you want to ramp up your vegetable intake, try dry vegetable powders in soups and smoothies. They're especially good for those who aren't that keen on actual vegetables. Super-easy and convenient with similar benefits as their non-powdered relatives.

GP *tip*

Don't waste leftover vegetables. Chop them up and throw them into pasta sauce or egg-fried rice, or even freeze them for later. They can have several chapters in their careers.

GP *tip*

Root vegetables absorb a lot from the soil in which they grow. That's why it's better to choose organic options wherever possible.

the totally-not-straightforward thing about fruit

Fruit... Well, it's a bit complicated. For the most part, it's very good for you because it contains lots of super-healthy antioxidants, vitamins, minerals and phytonutrients. It's helpful for maintaining hydration because it contains a lot of water. And the kind with edible skin is often a great source of soluble fibre. However, bear in mind that it can be pretty sugary, especially the particularly sweet, tropical kind, so focus on fruit with a low GL.

▸ **Low-GL fruit:** *Grapefruits, oranges, pears, peaches, apples, watermelon, strawberries, plums, blueberries, blackberries, dried apricots, cherries, prunes*

GP *tip*

Minimise the blood sugar spike by eating sweeter fruits with protein, like live natural yogurt, nuts and nut butter, seeds or even a piece of cheese.

GP *tip*

Ditch your shop-bought ice cream and make your own. Blitz up your favourite fruit with live natural yogurt or kefir (natural sugar and protein combo for the win) and freeze. Hello, healthy-digestion-friendly, free-from-E-numbers ice cream!

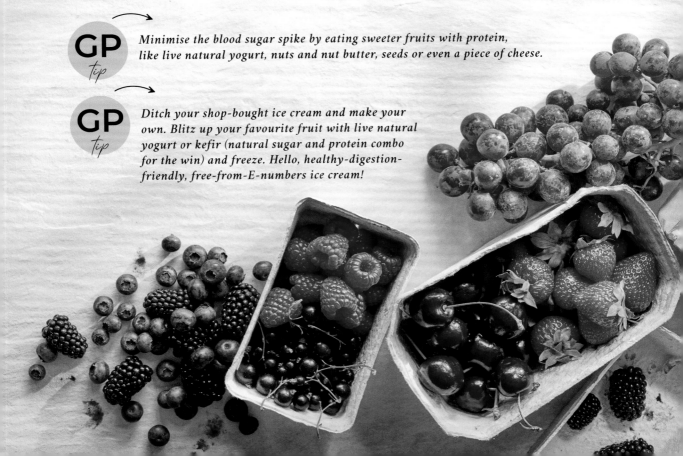

glorious grains

Grains are the seeds from cereal plants like rice and oats, and pseudo cereal plants like buckwheat and quinoa. Whole grains are nutrient A-graders, packed with fibre, iron, vitamin B, magnesium, phosphorus, selenium and manganese. They are a fantastic source of vegan protein and are lovely and filling – all of which is extremely helpful for healthy longevity. Yay!

Refined grains are the trouble-makers at the back of the class. Sometimes known as 'empty calories', these types of grains have had their goodness removed through processing, which basically turns them into a kind of simple sugar. Baaaaaad.

▶ **Wholegrains:** *oats, barley, millet, buckwheat, quinoa, brown rice, wild rice, whole wheat, whole rye, bulgar wheat, amaranth*

▶ **Refined grains:** *white-flour products (white bread, croissants, baguette), white rice, white pasta, pastries*

The general rule of thumb is: the darker and more you have to chew the bread, the better it is for you. It's that simple.

a really tiny note on bread

Bread is not the enemy, as some people believe. It just depends on what type. Anything dark and dense with seeds, nuts and grains – like pumpernickel or rye – is rich in nutrients. What you want to avoid is the white, processed kind that has resulted from mass production to meet years of growing demand. It calls itself bread, but it bears little resemblance to its healthier cousin.

Gluten or gluten-free? The answer is in the quality of the bread – whether it's gluten-free or not, processed is never better than a bread made from naturally gluten-free grains like quinoa, buckwheat or brown rice.

Crackers are an excellent alternative to bread, if you're in the mood for something satisfying but lighter – especially the kind with flaxseeds, which are high in fat and vegan protein. (There's even a handy recipe for these on page 133.)

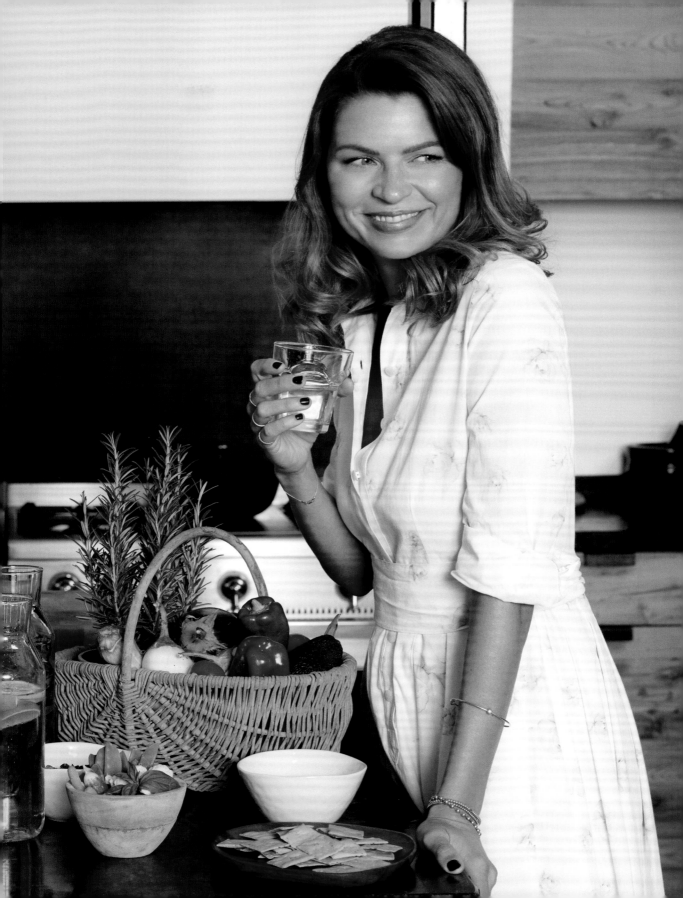

fun facts about fats

Fats play an incredibly important role in longevity. Research has shown that including a balance of fats from the top three categories in the diet is essential for numerous biochemical processes – and one of those happens to be increasing lifespan.

Coming mainly in the form of triglycerides, there are four fatty acid groups which contain different chemical structures and come from different sources. Triglycerides are large molecules composed of three fatty acid chains attached to glycerol. The differences in these chain attachments determines what function the fats themselves will play in the body and in what group they are identified. Within these groups, some fats are better than others, and knowing the difference makes all the difference. It's a common mistake to cut out fats when trying to lose weight; this often leaves the body feeling dissatisfied, which can lead to unhealthy cravings and bad habits.

As for fat-free foods – well! These processed products often use refined sugar to replace the removed fat, which can actually contribute to weight gain because the body is forced to store the excess sugar as triglycerides in fat cells. #shortlifespan

We need good fats. Cell membranes are largely comprised of lipids (glam word for a type of fat), which makes them essential for cell health. The body also relies on fats to absorb fat-soluble vitamins like A, D and E. Plus some essential fats are highly anti-inflammatory. #eternalyouth

gold medal: polyunsaturated fatty acids

These world-champion, record-breaking athletes of the fat world have been scientifically proven to increase longevity. The two main types of polyunsaturated fats are omega 3 and omega 6. These essential fatty acids are crucial for brain function, cell growth and cardiovascular health, among many other benefits. Regularly eating foods that contain both of them is vital, as they are the only fats the body cannot produce.

People tend to have higher levels of omega 6 in their diet – and while it has many beneficial elements, it can also increase inflammation. Omega 3, however, acts as a counterpart to omega 6, as it is packed with anti-inflammatory properties – in fact, studies have revealed that higher levels of omega 3 in the bloodstream have significantly impacted lifespan for the better.

▶ **Omega 3:**
Eat more fish (mackerel, herring, salmon, trout, sardines, tuna), shellfish (prawns, mussels, clams, crayfish, oysters), nuts (walnuts, almonds, macadamia nuts hazelnuts, pecans), seeds (pumpkin, sunflower, hemp, chia, flax)

▶ **Omega 6:**
Vegetable oils (safflower, sunflower, walnut, soybean)

Nuts and seeds: keep them in a jar on your kitchen counter and throw them on everything you eat. My work here is done.

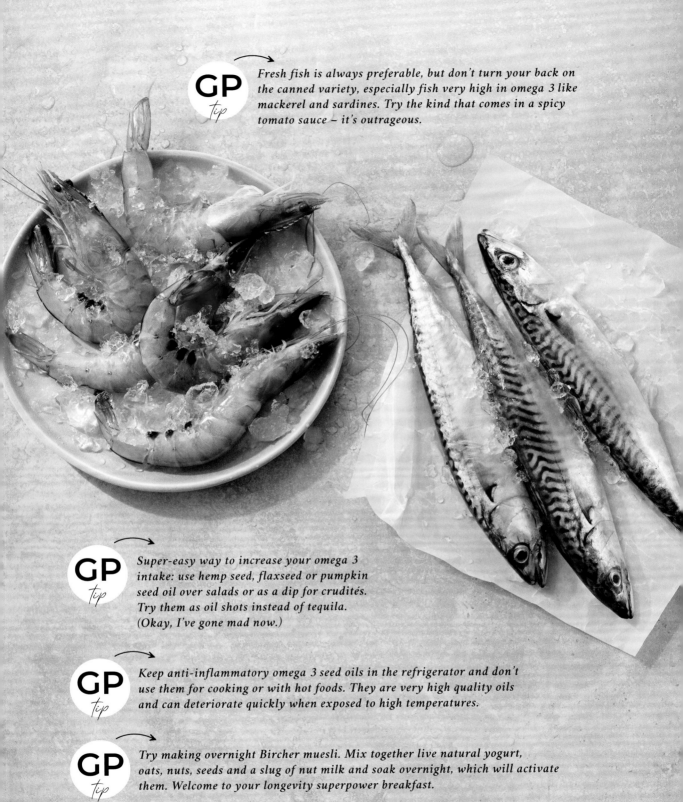

GP *tip*

Fresh fish is always preferable, but don't turn your back on the canned variety, especially fish very high in omega 3 like mackerel and sardines. Try the kind that comes in a spicy tomato sauce – it's outrageous.

GP *tip*

Super-easy way to increase your omega 3 intake: use hemp seed, flaxseed or pumpkin seed oil over salads or as a dip for crudités. Try them as oil shots instead of tequila. (Okay, I've gone mad now.)

GP *tip*

Keep anti-inflammatory omega 3 seed oils in the refrigerator and don't use them for cooking or with hot foods. They are very high quality oils and can deteriorate quickly when exposed to high temperatures.

GP *tip*

Try making overnight Bircher muesli. Mix together live natural yogurt, oats, nuts, seeds and a slug of nut milk and soak overnight, which will activate them. Welcome to your longevity superpower breakfast.

silver medal: monounsaturated fatty acids

In second place, we have monounsaturated fats, which have been shown to extend lifespan, as they reduce the risk of heart disease by improving insulin sensitivity, boosting immunity and supporting healthy weight loss. It's no coincidence that olive oil is a key component of the diet in the Mediterranean where they are living long and sprightly lives.

▸ **Monounsaturated fats:**
olive oil, avocados, nuts (almonds, cashew nuts, peanuts, pistachios), seeds (pumpkin, sunflower), eggs

Switch crisps for olives. The oleic acid in them activates longevity enzymes (even when they're added to martinis? I hope!)

Avocados are so versatile: use as a dairy fat substitute in ice cream and chocolate mousse or mix them with plenty of lime, coriander and chilli for guacamole.

bronze medal: saturated fats

The key to a successful relationship with saturated fats to not overdo it. Too much can ramp up cholesterol levels, but in moderation, saturated fats can help balance intestinal microflora and keep bones healthy, support the immune system and aid the liver in processing impurities. It's not uncommon for people to reduce their intake of saturated fats, but research has shown that we do need them for healthy longevity.

▸ **Saturated fats:**
fatty cuts of meat (lamb, pork, beef, dark poultry meat and skin), high-fat dairy (whole milk, butter, ghee, cheese, ice cream), coconut oil

When frying, swap oil for ghee, which has a higher smoke point and a delicious buttery taste. For some reverse-ageing house points, buy a variety mixed with turmeric (or just add it yourself).

Use coconut oil in smoothies or as your fat when baking. It works really well with sweet foods like cakes and cookies.

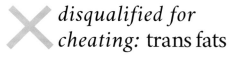

disqualified for cheating: trans fats

While some trans fats naturally occur in types of meat and dairy, it's the artificial kind you want to keep an eye out for. They run rife in processed foods in the form of hydrogenated and vegetable oils, as these help retain flavour and extend shelf life. Eat them once in a blue moon and you'll live. Eat them regularly and you're asking for trouble.

▸ **Trans fats:**
fried food (French fries, doughnuts, deep-fried fast foods), margarine, shop-bought baked goods (biscuits, cakes, pastries, pies), frozen pizza, processed snacks, hydrogenated vegetable oils

fantastic longevity-loving foods

The GP principles lay out the foundations for how to maximise food's effects on the body, but within that, certain food groups are professors in longevity – experts that specialise in everything from reducing inflammation to stimulating sirtuin enzymes, boosting antioxidant levels and balancing hormones. These foods are the gateway to increased energy and mental clarity, cheerful moods, better sleep, glowing skin and a healthy weight. The secret pathways to the fountain of youth. Like Edward Cullen, the hot vampire in *Twilight*.

sirtfoods: *the stress activators*

What do you mean you can't remember what sirtuins are? Are you not learning this book by heart? Okay, a little refresher – sirtuins are the specialised genes that are activated in response to hormesis, guarding against ageing and illness by repairing DNA and preserving genome integrity. Their effect on the body is similar to that of a calorie-restricted diet: mobilising stored fat, reducing inflammation, helping balance blood sugar levels and boosting energy by increasing mitochondrial function within the cell.

The thing about sirtfoods is that they come with a veritable circus of benefits, not just that they stimulate the production of sirtuin longevity enzymes. These plant-based foods can already boast that they are extremely healthy for the body, but they also contain longevity-stimulating phytonutrients called polyphenols.

Found especially in the skin, polyphenols are compounds in the edible parts of plans. They also give plants their colour (the darker, the better, just so you know), taste and smell. All this, and they're packed with antioxidants, vitamins and minerals.

Plants produce polyphenols in response to a threatening situation – maybe a bird is giving them the eye or a snail is licking its lips. When we eat plants that have produced this chemical stress response, we ingest those chemicals. They trigger a reaction in the body that makes it stronger and more resilient, with some especially stimulating sirtuin activity, thanks to the plant that had a really bad day.

▶ **Sirt foods:**
   Apples, citrus fruit (oranges, lemons, limes, grapefruits), strawberries, blueberries, Medjool dates, celery, capers, parsley, rocket, kale, red onions, chillies, red chicory, soya, buckwheat, walnuts, turmeric, extra virgin olive oil, green tea, red wine, cocoa (in the form of dark chocolate).

GP
tip

Summer cordial alert: juice some sirtuin-loving lemons or grapefruit into a bottle, add a squeeze of agave syrup and some sliced red chillies – add to sparkling water for a fresh and spicy metabolism booster.

Why have normal crisps when you could have sirtuin-stimulating, antioxidant/ polyphenol/vitamin/mineral and all-round youth-inducing kale chips? I even have a recipe for you on page 165. Chop! Chop!

 Look at your plate of food. How much colour is there? A simple trick is to think of the rainbow and include as many coloured foods as possible.

 Listen up. Frozen berries. Drenched in melted dark chocolate. Sirtuin-stimulation happening all over the place. Thank me later.

 Chopped red onion soaked in lemon juice slightly pickles it, reducing its pungency but adding to its sirtuin-stimulating capabilities. Add it to salads for a zingy crunch.

The trick when choosing dark chocolate is to go for one containing at least 70 per cent cocoa. This will ensure a high concentration of sirtuin stimulants and lower levels of sugar and dairy.

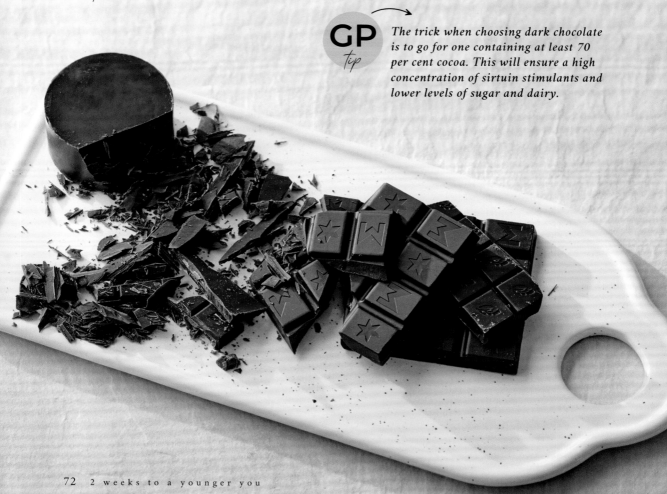

anti-inflammatory specialists

Chronic inflammation is one of the worst enemies of longevity. It can influence how the body gains weight, the development of biochemical imbalances and illnesses, energy and hormonal levels and sleep quality – everything from how you feel to how you look. Managing inflammation will therefore have a huge impact on how the body ages.

Fortunately, there are lots of different types of food with strong anti-inflammatory properties, and it's important to ensure your diet contains a broad mix of them, as they all play slightly different roles. Some of them specialise in immunity support, some in keeping the liver ship-shape, while others balance moods, increase energy and improve cognitive function – all of them are fantastic for general health, smoothing the path to longevity.

Herbs, herbs and more herbs. Rich in polyphenols, fresh herbs should be eaten as much as possible. A handy trick is to chop them up and store them in ice cube freezer trays to keep them fresh; defrost when needed.

▶ **Essential fatty acids:** *oily fish (salmon, mackerel, sardines), nuts (hazelnuts, cashew nuts, Brazil nuts, almonds, walnuts, macadamia nuts), seeds (pumpkin, sunflower, hemp, chia, flax), avocados*

▶ **Sulphurous foods:** *cruciferous vegetables (kale, cabbage, broccoli, Brussels sprouts, bok choy, cauliflower), alliums (onions, garlic, chives, shallots, leeks), eggs*

▶ **Red and purple fruit:** *blueberries, cherries, pomegranates, strawberries, blackberries, red grapes, raspberries, blackcurrants, cranberries*

▶ **Citrus fruits:** *lemons, limes, oranges, grapefruits, tangerines, satsumas, clementines, yuzu*

▶ **Super greens:** *green tea, matcha, wheatgrass, spirulina, chlorella*

▶ **Sprouted seeds and beans:** *lentils, chickpeas, alfalfa sprouts, broccoli, kale, radishes, mung beans*

▶ **Herbs and spices:** *ginger, turmeric, cinnamon, parsley, rosemary, garlic, cardamom, black pepper, ginseng, chillies, cloves*

Turmeric. The all-conquering anti-inflammatory master of the universe. Put it in literally everything – lattes, ghee, honey, nut butter, smoothies, soups – and laugh as your inflammation levels drop to their knees.

A little heads-up: if we're going to pick winners, berries and cantaloupe melon come out as the lowest in sugars, making them the best for healthy longevity. Get snacking.

GP tip

Sprouted grains or seeds, such as mung beans, broccoli, kale and alfalfa, are highly potent sources of activated goodness. Low in calories and incredibly rich in fibre, enzymes, protein, phytonutrients and micronutrients, they are like tiny nutrient explosions.

cooked? raw? frozen?

The best – and frankly most practical way – to eat phytonutrients is to mix it up. Many frozen vegetables and fruit retain their goodness very well, plus they are super-convenient, and we all need a bit of that.

The optimal way to cook vegetables is to steam them using a little bit of water, as boiling can zap them of their goodness. Steaming not only makes them easier to digest, it also increases their nutrient, vitamin and antioxidant availability. The key is to steam them until they're tender but still have their colour.

GP tip

Capsaicin is the anti-inflammatory ingredient found in the chilli pepper family that gives chillies their heat. If you don't like your chillies scorching hot, go for something milder like jalapeños, as you'll still get the benefits.

GP tip

Juice shots! These little concentrated pockets of goodness are quicker and less sugary than a full-sized juice. Try any combination of ginger, lemon, wheatgrass, parsley, celery and turmeric.

GP tip

Soak nuts and seeds overnight in water to activate their nutrient content and make them easier to digest.

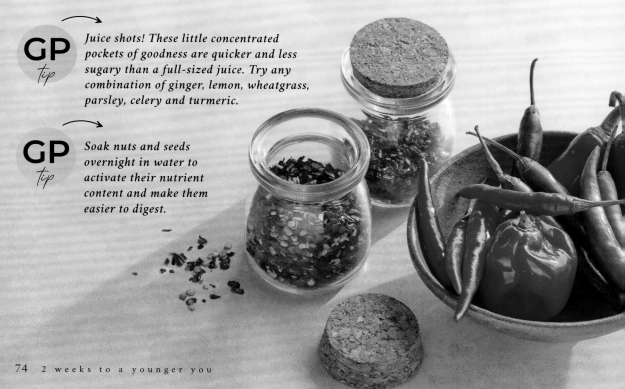

digestion and immunity cheerleaders

Nutrients and their powerful capabilities enter the body through digestion. This process needs to work seamlessly at every stage in order to break down, absorb and utilise nutrients to maximum effect – a healthy digestive system is the foundation on which multiple processes within the body depend in order to do their job.

To help every stage of digestion, munch down some bitter leaves like chicory or rocket as a starter, as they initiate the enzyme production in advance of what you eat next.

Within the digestive tract lies a magical kingdom of bacteria. Known as the intestinal microbiota (see page 47), this diverse community of microbes plays a key role in multiple functions within the body. One of the most important relationships it has is with the immune system. In fact, around 70 per cent of the body's immune system is housed in the digestive tract, fact fans.

Microbiota communicates closely with the central nervous system, which directly influences emotions and moods. It synthesizes nutrients like vitamins K and B, which are essential for energy production, and produces roughly 95 per cent of the body's serotonin – the 'happy' neurotransmitter. Serotonin plays integral roles in mental health, memory, sleep, digestion and appetite. It's the ultimate multi-tasker (must be a woman). Keep it onside all your life and you'll reap the rewards (also like a woman).

Miso makes you smile. Add seaweed to this microbiota-loving soup for an extra superfood kick. Keep a sachet in your bag and just add hot water for snacks on the run.

Rich in potassium, magnesium and calcium, bone broth can be home made from the bones of organic beef or the carcass of an organic chicken. A warm, soothing way to heal the intestinal lining and digestive tract.

the four 'R' protocol

The best way to balance digestive issues is to follow the four 'R' protocol.

1 remove

Identify triggers such as high sensitivity foods and reduce non-beneficial microbes.

- **Common suspects:** *eggs, gluten, dairy and grains; inflammatory foods (processed meat, refined carbohydrates, sugary foods and drinks, alcohol, trans fats); stress*

- **Banish non-beneficial microbes with spices and herbs:** *garlic, coriander, parsley, lemon grass, rosemary, cinnamon, cloves, sage and oregano*

GP *tip*
Keep your microbes friendly by eating plenty of garlic – let it sit for a few minutes after grating in order to activate its antimicrobial properties.

GP *tip*
If you have your suspicions, remove the food that you think might be triggering an issue and see if digestion improves. If not, keep going until you find the culprit.

2 replace

Support digestion by addressing any potential deficiencies, from low digestive enzyme levels, to low stomach acid.

- **Include bitter foods in your diet:** *rocket, radicchio, artichokes, chicory, dandelion greens, apple cider vinegar*

- **Choose supplements with digestive enzymes containing HCL** *(particularly with rich or protein-heavy meals)*

- **Experiment with bitter tonics:** *berberine, fennel seed, ginger, gentian, dandelion*

GP *tip*
Help break down food by drinking 2 tablespoons of apple cider vinegar mixed with a little bit of water before eating a protein-rich meal.

GP *tip*
Papaya and pineapple contain the enzymes papain and bromelain, which are natural digestive stimulants, making the fruits perfect for a light, outrageously healthy dessert.

3 reinoculate

Improve the balance of beneficial bacteria to restore healthy microbiota.

▶ **Increase your intake of prebiotics:** *leeks, onions, asparagus, bananas, garlic, artichokes, dandelion greens, agave, wheat bran, apples, strawberries, nuts (almonds, cashew nuts, walnuts), seeds (pumpkin, sunflower, hemp, chia, flax), psyllium, oats, celery, beans, lentils, peas*

▶ **And try probiotics:** *live natural yogurt, kefir, tofu, miso, kimchi, tempeh, kombucha, sauerkraut*

4 repair

Support the healing of the digestive tract to create a healthy environment.

▶ **L-glutamine foods:** *chicken, fish, spinach, cabbage, beans, tofu, lentils, dairy*

▶ **Omega 3:** *oily fish (salmon, mackerel, sardines), seeds (pumpkin, chia, flax), nuts (almonds, walnuts, hazelnuts)*

▶ **Phytonutrient champions:** *blueberries, blackberries, broccoli, red peppers, butternut squash, beetroot*

GP tip
Fire up good bacteria levels with probiotic supplements. Go for 10 billion CFU of a multi-strain variety for everyday digestive maintenance and increase to 30–50 billion CFU if you're experiencing imbalances of any kind.

GP tip
Kombucha has been gaining popularity over the past couple of years and is a really healthy alternative to soft drinks. With a massive range of different flavours, there is one out there for you. Believe.

GP tip
Beans are rich in digestion-loving fibre and vegan protein, and leave you feeling satisfied and full. Mix them with pasta – or get a bean variety of pasta – to balance blood sugar levels.

GP tip
Following a month of probiotics, restore the integrity of the intestine with these super-nutrient supplements: curcumin, slippery elm, aloe vera, deglycyrrhised liquorice, omega 3 and L-glutamine.

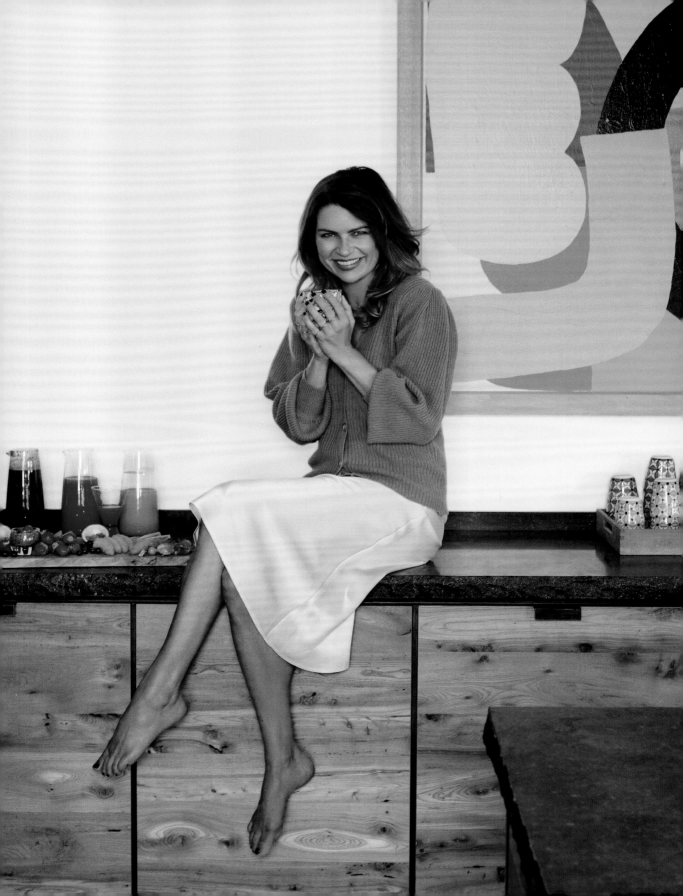

drink up

I can't overstate the importance of hydration. The body heavily depends on being hydrated to perform multiple functions, from flushing out impurities, nourishing the skin, supporting cognitive function and increasing energy levels to transporting oxygen, glucose and nutrients to cells, aiding digestion and keeping joints supple – all of which impact how the body ages.

water

Ensure you top up hydration levels throughout the day, particularly what is lost through sweat during hot weather, exercise, physical exertion and longevity-supporting activities like saunas. Apart from anything else, water regulates the body's cooling system. Make a habit of drinking regularly to help keep your internal rivers running nicely. Water really is the stuff of life.

Make water more interesting by steeping different flavours in a jug. Lemons, limes, mint, rosemary and cucumber are all delicious and will entice you to drink more.

how much do I need?

Drinking 1.5–2.5 litres (2.5–4.5 pints) of water throughout the day (this includes non-caffeinated beverages like herbal teas) is the average recommendation for most adults. Increase according to activity levels, if needed.

During particularly hot weather, replace lost electrolytes and increase hydration by adding a crystal or two of Himalayan pink salt to your water or by adding a sachet of rehydration powder.

Sorry to break the news, but fruit juices shouldn't count as part of your daily water intake purely because they're super-sweet. Apart from upsetting your blood sugar levels, they're quite calorific – but if you're really craving a freshly squeezed juice, mix it with water and I might turn a blind eye.

the two faces of caffeine

Caffeine can be something of a mixed bag, with its tendency to imbalance blood sugar levels. Having said that, caffeine-containing drinks like coffee and green tea come with lots of benefits, too. Caffeine can increase the body's metabolic rate and stimulate the nervous system, assist healthy weight loss by triggering the release of fatty acids from fat cells in adipose tissue, improve focus and elevate mood. Consuming moderate levels of caffeine while intermittent fasting can also help to ease cravings and keep energy levels buoyant.

When it comes to longevity, studies have revealed that regularly drinking coffee and tea can actually protect our DNA against neurodegeneration. And there's more. With high levels of antioxidants, notably the polyphenol chlorogenic acid, coffee's many bioactive substances deliver anti-inflammatory properties, reduce insulin resistance and protect against cell damage. Unite, caffeine drinkers of the world! Life is good.

► *Keep an eye on the amount of caffeine that you drink and try to always have it with a protein-rich snack or meal. However, during periods of IF, it's fine to bend this rule a little if you are in real need of a pick-me-up.*

► *Make sure that any caffeinated drinks consumed during IF do not contain any dairy or nut milk, as they will interfere with the efficiency of autophagy.*

► *The effects of caffeine play out differently for everyone, with some people finding they can tolerate much more than others. Understand how it works for you, so that you can reap the rewards of the benefits and dial down the negative effects.*

GP *tip*

Rooibos (red bush) is a deliciously fragrant alternative to caffeinated tea – plus it's packed with antioxidants and is one of the only herbal teas to which you can add milk. You might not even notice the difference.

a little note on MCTs

MCT (Medium Chain Triglycerides) molecules are lipids, naturally occurring in substances like coconut oil and dairy products, but also available as a concentrated oil or powder. Their shorter chains mewn they are quickly digested, and they are converted into ketones rather than stored as fat, making them an immediate source of energy. Benefits include increasing physical stamina, improved feelings of satiety and sharper mental clarity.

GP
tip

Green tea and matcha are my favourite caffeinated teas because they come with a veritable party bag of sirtuin stimulants and longevity-supporting antioxidants. Watch yourself get younger as you drink them.

GP
tip

Try adding MCT powder to coffee or tea instead of milk. You'll feel fuller for longer, be able to exercise for longer, stay cleverer for longer, have balanced blood sugar levels for longer, live longer...

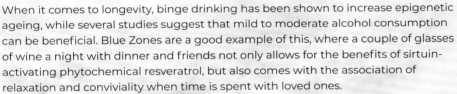

alcohol. It's good news...

I'm not really in a position to tell people to put down the bottle. I love a good glass of wine (maybe more than my children – don't tell them I said that), but if I'm going to be boring, then yes, alcohol is not without its negatives. It's sugary, full of empty calories and puts extra strain on the liver if you overdo it. This impacts the equilibrium of the body and negatively affects the immune system, digestion, mood, sleep and energy levels. Plus too much of it too often can make you put on weight, typically around the midriff. On the plus side – it's fun! And it tastes nice! And it makes boring people more interesting! And makes us more interesting! Or not! Who cares because we're drunk!

When it comes to longevity, binge drinking has been shown to increase epigenetic ageing, while several studies suggest that mild to moderate alcohol consumption can be beneficial. Blue Zones are a good example of this, where a couple of glasses of wine a night with dinner and friends not only allows for the benefits of sirtuin-activating phytochemical resveratrol, but also comes with the association of relaxation and conviviality when time is spent with loved ones.

GP
tip

Mixers are usually sugary and will ramp up the calorie intake, so avoid where possible. If you're desperate for something sweet in your drink, try kombucha, flavoured sparkling waters or coconut water.

GP
tip

Spirits like vodka, gin and tequila are best when they're diluted, so have them with ice or sparkling water. Add a spritz or slice of lemon or lime to give your liver a helping hand.

GP
tip

To really boost resveratrol levels (which would take more wine than even I could drink), try taking it in supplement form at a recommended dose of 250–500mg daily.

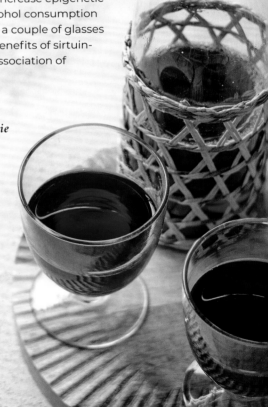

the GP intermittent fasting longevity plans

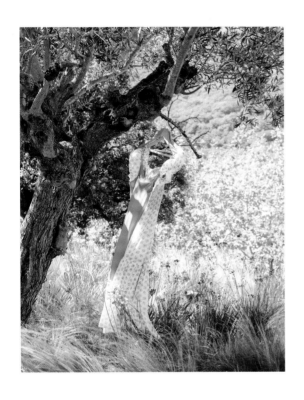
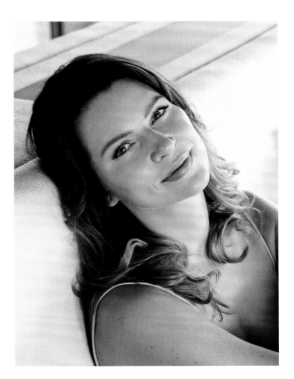
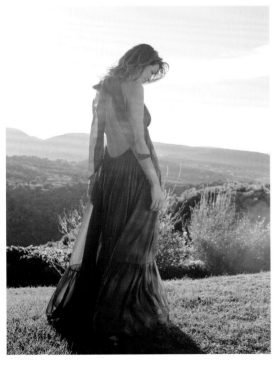
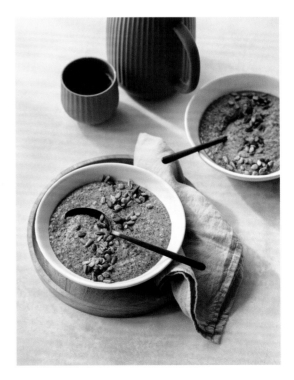

RIGHT. So let's actually do this. Intermittent fasting (IF) is scientifically proven to work. I've seen it for myself, over and over again. It's the easiest, most sustainable way to lose weight and recharge the body. Apart from healthy weight loss, the effects are incredible, from transforming sleep, energy levels and mental clarity, to boosting immunity – and that's before we've even talked about its impact on longevity.

The anti-ageing capabilities of IF are making real waves in the scientific world. Ongoing research is revealing more and more information about how the effects of hormetic stress, the stimulation of autophagy and the radical clearing of senescent cells (longevity's greatest enemy) is disrupting the ageing process by slowing it down and profoundly recalibrating how the body behaves. IF allows you to take back control of your body – and what's amazing is that you'll feel the difference quickly. The psychological impact of this plays a huge role in the success of IF, which is just as important as the physical effects. When you can feel the changes and understand why they're happening, it's very empowering. You've put yourself back in charge – and it feels great.

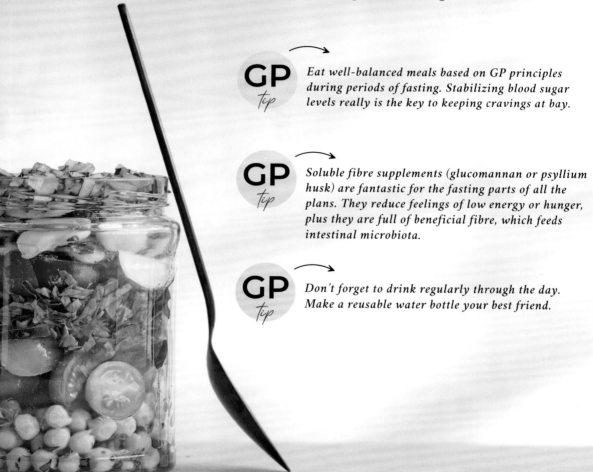

GP *tip*

Eat well-balanced meals based on GP principles during periods of fasting. Stabilizing blood sugar levels really is the key to keeping cravings at bay.

GP *tip*

Soluble fibre supplements (glucomannan or psyllium husk) are fantastic for the fasting parts of all the plans. They reduce feelings of low energy or hunger, plus they are full of beneficial fibre, which feeds intestinal microbiota.

GP *tip*

Don't forget to drink regularly through the day. Make a reusable water bottle your best friend.

which plan to choose?

When it comes to choosing a plan*, it's important to be honest with yourself about which one will work for you. It's absolutely fine to experiment and see which one lands, as you're far more likely to stick to something that feels convenient, achievable and fits in with your lifestyle. We are all biologically unique with different goals, which is why I have prepared three options to choose from.

I recommend having a read through each plan before you begin and go from there. Starting any kind of new programme can feel a little daunting, but I can guarantee two things: they will work, and you will feel completely transformed.

These plans are recommended for adults with no significant medical health conditions, and a healthy BMI. It is always recommended before making any dietary changes or starting any weight loss plans to consult your doctor or other health professional.

introducing the two-week IF plans

SUPER-CHARGE 700	RESET 700	LIVE LONG 16:8
Most restrictive programme for targeted and significant healthy weight loss, cellular cleansing and transformed biochemistry	A less restrictive programme for increased longevity, resetting the body's systems and healthy weight loss	The mildest programme, ideal for less significant weight loss or maintaining a healthy weight, while still improving longevity
16:8 with focus on GP principles	**16:8** with focus on GP principles	**16:8** with focus on the GP principles
WEEK 1: 24-hour fast	**WEEK 1:** *Optional* 24-hour fast	**WEEK 1:** *Optional* 24-hour fast
Three consecutive days of 700 calories maximum	Two consecutive days of 700 calories maximum	No specific calorie restriction but mindful eating
WEEK 2: Repeat	**WEEK 2:** Repeat	**WEEK 2:** All mindful days

SUPER-CHARGE 700

This plan delivers the biggest changes. Starting with a 24-hour fast, it sends the body into a state of turbo-charged autophagy.

Three days of low-calorie intake follow, which allow your body to make amazing changes by clearing out redundant particles of cells, significantly upgrading cellular activity and starting to use energy more efficiently while keeping mTOR levels low. This, along with having a time-restricted eating window during the two weeks of 16:8, will keep the body in a deficit state, driving it to deplete excess fat reserves, which will lead to healthy weight loss.

Like going to the gym or taking up running for the first time, any change can be daunting. But once you start, you may well find it's not as challenging as you thought it was going to be – and remember, amazing transformations are happening inside your body.

To keep autophagy fully activated over the three 700-calorie days, I recommend choosing vegan options over animal protein, particularly low-calorie soups and salads. There are lots of ideas in the recipes section, as well as snacks. You're not going to evaporate into a mist.

RESET 700

Still highly effective, this is a slightly gentler version of the Super-charge 700 plan and is a good one to start with if you've never tried fasting or time-restricted eating before.

The optional 24-hour fast, followed by two days of 700 calories and 16:8 time-restricted eating will still render significant results, but might be psychologically a bit easier initially. My patients often find that once they know what calorie-restricted days are like, it's easier to extend to three days the following week – but it's fine if you'd rather stick to just two.

As with the first plan, it's important to stay within the 700-calorie restriction and to go for vegan options over animal protein to keep the body in a state of autophagy, as well as to trigger it to burn fat reserves as a source of energy.

With effects that are similar to the Super-charge 700 plan, the Reset 700 plan is a great option for better sleep, increased energy and improved longevity by clearing redundant cells and regenerating new ones. Think of it as a spring clean for healthy ageing with the added benefit of weight loss.

Olives and nuts, with plenty of healthy fats, antioxidants and polyphenols, make great protein-rich vegan snacks during 700-calorie days. Ideal for taking the edge off cravings.

Contrary to what you might think, it's much better to keep busy during periods of fasting and 700-calorie days. Not only is the distraction helpful, the effects of fasting can make the brain feel sharper than normal, so you might even find you're more productive.

LIVE LONG
16:8

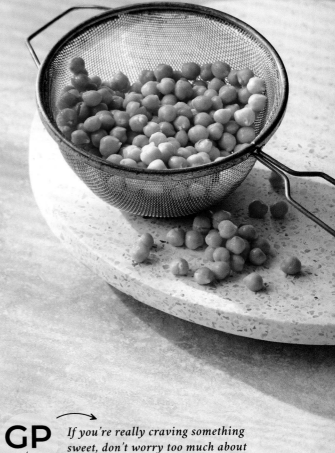

The 16:8 Live Long plan is a very popular intermittent fasting plan.

Time-restricted eating is backed by a lot of scientific research and has been widely proven to reset and upgrade the body's systems. It's also the easiest plan to fit in with your lifestyle, as the eight-hour eating window is flexible in terms of when you want to apply it each day. The 16-hour fast can predominantly be done overnight, which makes it a whole lot easier, as you're asleep for a large part of it.

While this plan does not involve specific calorie restriction like the other two, it does involve following the GP principles and eating mindfully. People tend to skip a meal in order to fit within the eight-hour eating window and this in itself reduces calorie intake. Levels of autophagy and weight loss are milder, but they're both still happening. The option to kick-start the plan with a 24-hour fast is up to you.

I've been recommending this plan for a decade and all my patients felt fantastic when they finished it. Easy and sustainable, it's incredibly good for you; and people commonly adopt it as a way of life, from extending the two weeks further to incorporating it into a handful of days a week. 16:8 is a healthier way to eat that your body will absolutely love.

GP *tip*
If you're really craving something sweet, don't worry too much about occasionally treating yourself. Try nuts, seeds or chickpeas covered in dark chocolate or some dried fruits – just don't go crazy.

GP *tip*
Starting your eight-hour eating window at different times during the 16:8 days during your plan is completely fine. It's all about flexibility and what you feel works best within the structure of your day.

GP *tip*
Choosing vegan protein and high-fibre vegetables during 700-calorie days will keep you in an autophagy state for longer. Yes please to all the tofu!

a little note on the 24-hour fast

These three plans are incredibly effective, but my clinical experience along with extensive scientific research shows that the hormetic effect of fasting completely for 24 hours will turbo-charge autophagy in the body in preparation for the following two weeks. Some people find it easier than others, but I really recommend trying it because it gives the body a complete break from digestion. The body will go into a temporary state of 'emergency', as the lack of fuel will drive it to source its energy from reserved stores – and this is where the magic happens.

Bone broths, soups, or any kind of light, cooked vegetable dishes are gentle, nourishing but low-calorie foods to introduce after fasting. This will also help keep autophagy going for longer.

It's not for everyone, but bowel cleansing during the 24-hour fast really increases its benefits. Try booking a colonic, or mix 1 teaspoon of internal-use Epsom salts (NOT the bath salts!) into a glass of warm water and drink.

Am I really hungry or am I just breaking a habit?

We form habits around the things we do at the same time every day – like eating – so disrupting what the body is used to on a daily basis will inevitably require a bit of adjusting. It's normal to worry a little about how you might feel during a more prolonged fast, but don't be discouraged if you feel hungry at points during the day. The hunger will subside as you adapt to a new eating pattern. Trust that your body knows what it's doing and that amazing things are happening beneath the surface.

Coffee and black tea is okay if you feel you need a bit of a brain-sharpening pick-me-up – just make sure you don't include milk as this will interfere with autophagy.

My favourite way of starting a 24-hour fast is to stop eating after supper on a Sunday night (this may or may not have to do with long, boozy weekend lunches – I'm saying nothing) so that I wake up the next morning knowing I can eat again that evening. Also, I will have slept through part of it, which makes the whole thing a lot easier.

24-hour fast advice

24 hours can feel like a long time – and in an ideal world, it's what you should aim for. Do the best you can, but don't panic if you find you need to build up to it. I do recommend trying to go for longer, but anything over 16 hours is good. Trust your body.

FREQUENTLY ASKED QUESTIONS

How can I expect to feel during the 24-hour fast?
It's normal to feel hungry, of course, and experience the side effects that can come with that (feeling a little bit moody or low on energy – you know the drill), but these feelings usually come and go. Your body is likely to adapt quicker than you might think.

If the 24-hour fast works for me, can I repeat it again in week two of the plan?
Yes! Feel free to repeat the fast again in the second week.

Should anyone not fast?
Fasting is only suitable for adults with a healthy BMI. Anyone with an ongoing medical condition or taking any kind of medication should consult their doctor or health professional first.

Can I do the 24-hour fast and still work as normal?
Absolutely. People think fasting means they collapse in a heap, but being busy actually makes it easier. Your body knows what it's doing and will support you through it.

Can I exercise?
This is a personal choice, but I would strongly recommend listening to your body. If the exercise doesn't feel good, stop. The body is in a temporary state of stress, so it's important not to push it. If you start fasting regularly, this may change as your body adapts, but in the early days, proceed with caution. If you love exercise, you could do some gentle forms of yoga and Pilates.

What if I want to stop?
If the 24-hour fast is not for you, that's okay. Don't feel too disheartened – you can continue with the rest of the plan as normal.

What should I eat once my 24-hour fast is over?
A light, easily digestible meal such as steamed vegetables, soup, soft foods like avocado or hummus with crackers (but not raw vegetables, as they are a little harder to digest).

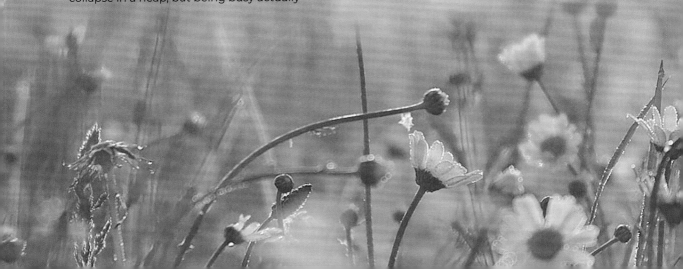

700 day advice

What to eat
Follow the GP eating principles and make sure you don't exceed 700 calories per day. Healthy meal composition will help prevent cravings, so try to incorporate:
- *High-fibre carbohydrates, especially non-starchy vegetables, as they are low in calories and will help you feel fuller for longer*
- *Vegetarian sources of protein, to maintain autophagy on these particular days*
- *Avoid high-fat foods like oil, butter and cheese as they will bring up your calorie count*

Counting calories
Your total daily calorie intake should be 700 or below during your designated days. There are lots of suggestions in the recipe section of this book (see pages 122–205), plus it's easy to search the internet for calorific information about the food you want to eat. Some people also find calorie tracking apps helpful, as they do the calculation for you. Hurray for anything that makes life easier.

Nutrient distribution
Distribute your calorie allowance according to what suits you, whether that's two or three small meals or one meal and a couple of snacks. Just try to space them out within your eight-hour eating window.

FREQUENTLY ASKED QUESTIONS

Do my 700-calorie days need to be consecutive?
Yes. It's important to keep the calories low on consecutive days because this will both activate and maintain autophagy.

What happens if I go a little bit over 700 calories?
It's not the end of the world if you exceed it by 50–100 calories, but more than that and you'll need to repeat the 700-calorie restriction the next day.

What if I eat less than 700 calories?
I don't recommend going below 700 calories on more than one day, but we are all different and this will depend on your age, health status, activity levels and if you're carrying excess weight.

Can I drink alcohol?
Alcohol is sugary and has calories in it, so I recommend cutting back. If you do have a drink, it needs to be during the eight-hour eating window.

What about caffeine?
Yes, it's fine – although don't have any milk in your drink outside the eight-hour eating window, as it counts as food.

Can I exercise?
Yes, it's fine to exercise – in fact, it has been shown to help the body enter a state of autophagy and ketosis more quickly – but as always, listen to your body.

How much weight will I lose during these plans?
This is completely individual and will depend on your starting weight, how closely you stick to a plan and your levels of physical activity. IF plans are designed to work with the body's innate intelligence to lose weight safely and sustainably.

mindful day advice

Follow the GP principles for healthy eating, stick to the eight-hour eating window and aim for your meals to be approximately 20 per cent smaller than normal. Alternatively, you could reduce your overall calorie intake by 20 per cent with a normal-size breakfast and/or lunch, finishing with a light supper.

And remember, this part of the plan does not involve calorie restriction to the same degree, so enjoy what you eat as long as it's healthy and balanced, for example:

- ► ½ *non-starchy vegetables (kale, spinach, broccoli), beans, courgettes*
- ► ¼ *wholegrains (brown rice, quinoa, barley) or starchy vegetables (potatoes, corn, peas)*
- ► ¼ *protein (fish, poultry, tofu, lean meat, dairy)*

FREQUENTLY ASKED QUESTIONS

Do I have to stick to the same times for my eight-hour eating window?
No – you can decide when you start the eating window each day.

Can I exercise?
Yes, exercise helps to improve longevity and burn calories more efficiently. See pages 108–110 for recommendations.

Can I drink alcohol?
Yes, but as it contains calories, keep it to within the eight-hour eating window.

Can I do the 16:8 plan for longer than two weeks?
Yes – it's a really healthy way of eating, so you can do it indefinitely, as long as you're a healthy weight.

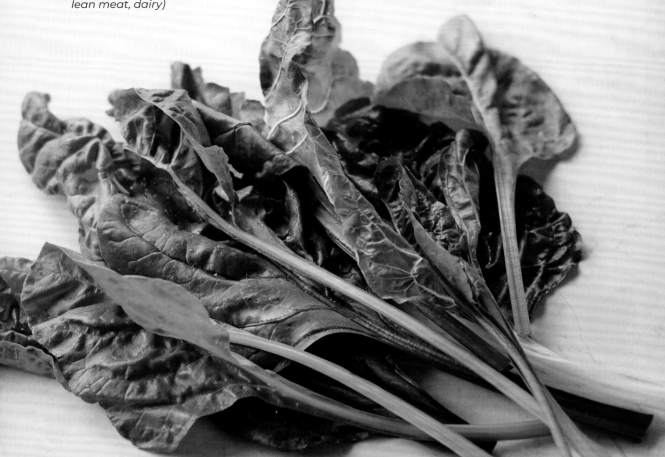

two-week **super-charge** 700 plan

DAY 1	24-hour fast	16:8	Water / herbal teas / black coffee / black tea
DAY 2	700 calories	16:8	Vegan or low animal protein
DAY 3	700 calories	16:8	Vegan or low animal protein
DAY 4	Mindful	16:8	GP principles
DAY 5	Mindful	16:8	GP principles
DAY 6	Mindful	16:8	GP principles
DAY 7	Mindful	16:8	GP principles
DAY 8	700 calories *OR* 24-hour fast	16:8	Vegan or low animal protein Water / herbal teas / black coffee / black tea
DAY 9	700 calories	16:8	Vegan or low animal protein
DAY 10	700 calories	16:8	Vegan or low animal protein
DAY 11	Mindful	16:8	GP principles
DAY 12	Mindful	16:8	GP principles
DAY 13	Mindful	16:8	GP principles
DAY 14	Mindful	16:8	GP principles

two-week **reset** 700 plan

DAY 1	700 calories *OR* 24-hour fast	16:8	Vegan or low animal protein Water / herbal teas / black coffee / black tea
DAY 2	700 calories	16:8	Vegan or low animal protein
DAY 3	Mindful	16:8	GP principles
DAY 4	Mindful	16:8	GP principles
DAY 5	Mindful	16:8	GP principles
DAY 6	Mindful	16:8	GP principles
DAY 7	Mindful	16:8	GP principles
DAY 8	700 calories *OR* 24-hour fast	16:8	Vegan or low animal protein Water / herbal teas / black coffee / black tea
DAY 9	700 calories	16:8	Vegan or low animal protein
DAY 10	Mindful	16:8	GP principles
DAY 11	Mindful	16:8	GP principles
DAY 12	Mindful	16:8	GP principles
DAY 13	Mindful	16:8	GP principles
DAY 14	Mindful	16:8	GP principles

two-week **live long** 16:8 plan

DAY 1	Mindful *OR* 24-hour fast	16:8	GP Principles Water / herbal teas / black coffee / black tea
DAY 2	Mindful	16:8	GP principles
DAY 3	Mindful	16:8	GP principles
DAY 4	Mindful	16:8	GP principles
DAY 5	Mindful	16:8	GP principles
DAY 6	Mindful	16:8	GP principles
DAY 7	Mindful	16:8	GP principles
DAY 8	Mindful	16:8	GP principles
DAY 9	Mindful	16:8	GP principles
DAY 10	Mindful	16:8	GP principles
DAY 11	Mindful	16:8	GP principles
DAY 12	Mindful	16:8	GP principles
DAY 13	Mindful	16:8	GP principles
DAY 14	Mindful	16:8	GP principles

planning your eight-hour eating window

EARLY BIRDS: If you prefer not to miss breakfast, eat in the morning and finish your eating window in the late afternoon. I recommend going to bed early to avoid feeling hungry in the evening.

Wake up–10am (FASTING)	8am–4pm (8-hour eating window)	4pm–Bedtime (FASTING)
WAKE UP Morning part of your 16-hour fast	10am: first meal 1pm: snack/small meal 5pm: last meal	Evening part of your 16-hour fast **GO TO BED**

MIDDLE-OF-THE-DAY-BIRDS: If you're happy to skip breakfast and prefer to have lunch and dinner at a more usual time, start at midday.

Wake up–12pm (FASTING)	12pm–8pm (8-hour eating window)	8pm–Bedtime (FASTING)
WAKE UP Morning part of your 16-hour fast	12pm: first meal 3.30pm: snack/small meal 7pm: last meal	Evening part of your 16-hour fast **GO TO BED**

NIGHT OWLS: With a slightly later lunch and extending the eating window into the evening. This is the best option for those who have evening engagements.

Wake up–2pm (FASTING)	2pm–10pm (8-hour eating window)	10pm–Bedtime (FASTING)
WAKE UP Morning part of your 16-hour fast	2pm: first meal 5pm: snack/small meal 9pm: last meal	Evening part of your 16-hour fast **GO TO BED**

longevity triggers

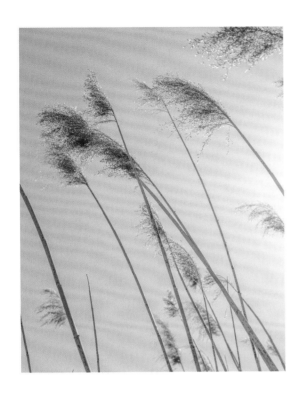
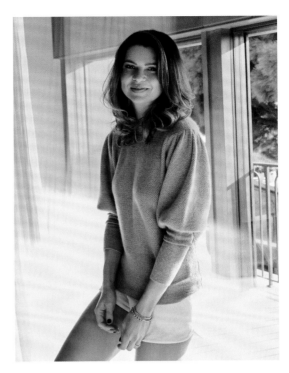
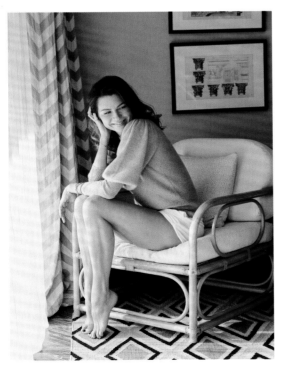
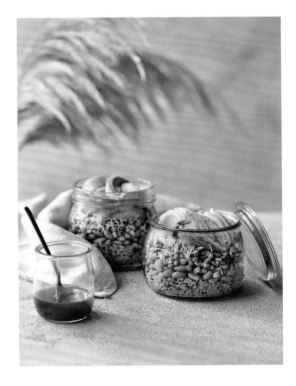

1 release the shock proteins:
the miraculous benefits of hot and cold therapy

Time to activate your heat-shock proteins, cold-shock proteins, protective brown fat and longevity genes! If you're backing away towards the door, don't worry – I'm talking about short, controlled exposures, not the extreme version where you sit in your underwear in a snowdrift.

Standing in a freezing shower for two minutes, swearing (at me?) might initially sound unappealing, but it's not going to ruin your day. Nor is sweltering in a steam room. Don't forget, these treatments are designed to put your body in a temporary state of stress. It lasts as long as you want it to last – but just know that your body and mind can and will adapt.

You may find that you prefer one to the other. You may also find that your body begins to respond to it even if your mind at first doesn't. Heat- or cold-shock therapy can be an extraordinary experience and there's a real sense of achievement that comes with doing either of them – plus the health benefits are off the scale. Increased energy, glowing skin, blood pumping, an invigorated mind, all wrapped up with an improved-longevity bow. Those are worth jumping into the cold sea for five minutes, right?

As with everything recommended in this book, don't push yourself too hard and always use common sense. If you have any questions or concerns, it's a good idea to chat them through with your GP (your doctor, still not me) first.

- ▶ Don't be afraid of being cold. Anything from exercising outdoors in winter to sleeping with fewer covers helps to build resilience.

- ▶ Start small by alternating the temperature in your shower. Try 1–2 minutes of cold water, then switch to warm water for the same amount of time. Do this for a few rounds to increase blood flow and fire up the lymphatic system.

- ▶ Progress to 10–15 minutes in a sauna or steam room, followed by jumping into a cold plunge pool or taking a cold shower for 1–2 minutes. It's important to repeat this three or four times in a row so the body doesn't adapt too quickly.

- ▶ Try cryotherapy, which involves exposing the body to extremely cold air in an enclosed chamber for a few minutes. It has incredible longevity-related benefits that include reducing inflammation and stress – plus it leaves the body stimulated and re-energised.

- ▶ Cold water swimming and ice baths are more extreme but even more rewarding, which is partly why they have become so popular. See how long you can last, but remember take it easy – your body needs to adjust, and the benefits come even from short exposure.

For a gentler experience, an infrared sauna is a great way to activate heat-shock proteins. Because the heat is considerably lower, you can stay in it for longer (maybe take a book with you – it's outrageously relaxing).

 To get the most out of the sauna-cold shower combo, try doing it no more than three or four times a week. Any more than that will reduce the effect of the hormetic stress, as your body may become too used to it.

 Keep hydration levels topped up by drinking plenty of water – for a healthy electrolyte boost, try diluted coconut water or a dash of fresh juice with a couple of Himalayan salt crystals in your water bottle.

 Dry brushing your body while in the sauna will get your lymphatic system moving, helping to support healthy immunity with the added bonus of making your skin look shiny and glowing.

2 time for bed: *sleep and re-energise*

The power of a good night's sleep goes beyond feeling cheerful in the morning – it's actually essential for our general health. A huge amount of housekeeping goes on within the body overnight, which is reliant on sleep quality. Sleep affects every area of physiological function in the body, from cellular renewal within the brain, muscles and organs, to healthy weight maintenance, hormone regulation and metabolic balancing. Continuously sleeping badly can profoundly impact not only general health but also how the body ages. Scientific research has shown that poor sleep can actually reduce life expectancy.

One of the most crucial ways to maintain the brain's and body's energy levels as the years progress is to keep the mitochondria – the battery of every cell – healthy and sparkly. It's not uncommon for mitochondria to start to wane and this decline is typically associated with cellular senescence (see page 19), inflammation and metabolic issues. Inevitably, this will enormously affect energy levels throughout the day, impacting productivity, enthusiasm for tasks, focus, work, happiness, mental health... (we could be here all day).

Along with keeping mitochondria fired up and energised, the hormone melatonin, which balances the circadian rhythm, also contributes to the regulation of autophagy by protecting the process with its antioxidant capabilities. It's essential to keep melatonin balanced and sleep rituals healthy in order to amplify energy levels, and there are lots of ways to do this.

Put your phone to sleep at night. Research suggests that EMF (electromagnetic field) exposure can disrupt melatonin secretion, so give yourself and your phone the night off by switching it off.

 Doing gentle yoga and meditation before bed are good ways to calm a racing brain, allowing the mind to separate itself from a busy day.

Good bedtime habits

▶ Try to go to bed and wake up at a similar time every day to regulate the circadian rhythm. This will support the brain to understand when it should be asleep and when it should be awake, helping to maximise melatonin production. It really helps to form a nightly bedtime ritual, from taking a bath to reading.

▶ Keep your bedroom cool to allow the body's core temperature to drop. This is essential to fall asleep – and stay asleep. Have the window open so fresh air can circulate, and make sure the room is dark.

▶ Try to stop looking at screens before bedtime. The blue light they emit can trick the brain into believing that it is, in fact, daytime, which prohibits the release of melatonin needed to help the body fall asleep.

▶ Being physically active in the day can help balance the body's energy levels and increase the desire to sleep. Just no HiiT classes right before bedtime.

▶ If you're feeling particularly stressed or busy, keep a notebook next to your bed to write down any thoughts circulating in your head and keeping you awake. There's something about externalising anxieties that can help you detach from them until morning.

 Blue light blocking glasses are the answer if you're obsessed with reality TV and you have to know if that couple will get together or be dumped from the island last thing at night.

 During hot summer evenings when the heat can make it harder to sleep, try putting a hot water bottle filled with cold water into the freezer for half an hour and then snuggling that instead of your annoying boiling hot bed companion.

sleep nutrient kings

GP *tip*
Keep blood sugar levels balanced throughout the day by eating regularly and including protein with every meal to maintain a healthy circadian rhythm that ends with a good night's sleep.

GP *tip*
Don't overeat late in the evening. Going to sleep on a full stomach can be uncomfortable and prevent the body from winding down – giving it half a cow to digest is not going to help you drift off.

MAGNESIUM

Magnesium comes out on top as the sleep nutrient to rule them all. Nature's relaxant, it does numerous jobs around the body, including reducing anxiety, stress and high blood pressure, which can deplete the levels that are needed for restful sleep. Magnesium deficiency is a common problem, so increasing intake can have amazing results.

▶ **Magnesium-rich foods**: *dark leafy greens (kale, spinach, chard, cavolo nero),* nuts (almonds, hazelnuts, cashew nuts, walnuts), seeds (pumpkin, sunflower, chia, hemp), grains (buckwheat, quinoa), beans, chickpeas, lentils, dark chocolate (70 per cent cocoa and above)

▶ *Soak in a bath of magnesium chloride flakes for at least 20 minutes before bedtime.*

▶ *Take magnesium supplements after dinner to help the body start to wind down as you head towards bedtime.*

GP *tip*
If you find you need to take magnesium in a higher dosage and you don't want to crunch down a fistful of tablets, try it in powder form mixed with a little water or spoonful of live natural yogurt.

GP *tip*
Magnesium partnered with glycinate or malate are the best supplement combinations to take, as they increase absorption.

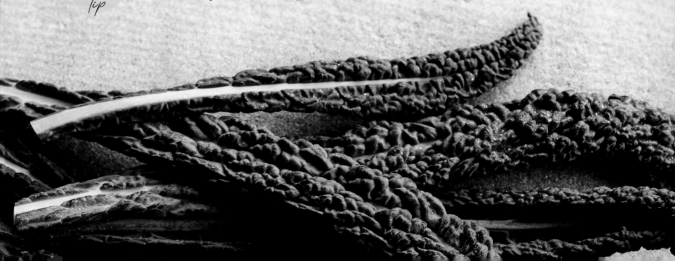

TRYPTOPHAN

Tryptophan is also a big winner when it comes to super-powered sleep nutrients. Found in protein, this amino acid helps the body sleep restfully as it's a precursor of serotonin, the 'happy' neurotransmitter that helps calm the brain.

▶ dairy products, poultry (turkey, chicken), peanuts, pumpkin seeds, sesame seeds, |eggs

Have a sneaky tryptophan snack before bed: a slice of turkey, or a couple of spoonfuls of cottage cheese or live natural yogurt will help you sleep.

Remember meal composition rules: a balance of protein (always protein), healthy fats and fibre-rich carbs, preferably the phytonutrient-packed colourful kind to sleep well and stay energised.

Don't be fooled by that lazy feeling. Sometimes it's a good idea to push yourself when you feel low on energy. Even though you might not feel like it when you're tired, walking around the block for ten minutes will leave you feeling surprisingly sprightly.

Charge up your energy

▶ Sugar is mean and so are refined carbohydrates, so eat less of both. They will trick you with their evil ways by making you briefly feel great before throwing your energy levels down in a surprise ninja move to leave you craving more.

▶ It is essential to keep blood sugar levels stable to prevent cravings, mood swings and energy dips, so ensure all meals are well composed according to the GP principles.

▶ Apart from stimulating a cellular spring clean through autophagy, IF specifically targets redundant or old mitochondria through mitophagy, which stimulates the growth of new mitochondria, boosts cellular function and increases energy levels.

▶ Exercising regularly is one of the best ways to stop feeling sluggish. Your body will generate more energy according to the energy you use.

energy nutrient queens

B VITAMINS

It's common for a lack of B vitamins to be the source of low energy, as they are some of the key players in helping the body's energy production cycle and metabolism. Keep them topped up to replace feelings of fatigue with increased focus and boosted vitality.

▶ **Plant sources:** *leafy green vegetables (kale, spinach, chard, cavolo nero, spring greens), wholegrains (buckwheat, brown rice, rye), beans (chickpeas, cannellini beans, kidney beans, black beans)*

▶ **Animal sources:** *fish (salmon, tuna, mackerel), shellfish (prawns, mussels, clams, oysters), eggs, dairy*

If you're feeling sluggish, I find a good B vitamin complex is far better than artificial energy drinks. Just ensure you take them with food, and then spring off into your day.

IRON AND IODINE

Iron is essential to the production of red blood cells. When iron levels are depleted, it impacts red blood cells' ability to deliver oxygen needed for the body's other cells to process glucose and generate energy.

▶ **Animal sources:** *lean red meat (beef, lamb, pork), seafood (oysters, scallops, mussels, clams)*

▶ **Plant sources:** *beans and pulses (soya beans, kidney beans, butterbeans, chickpeas, lentils), leafy greens (kale, chard, spinach), nuts (almonds, hazelnuts, cashew nuts, macadamia nuts), seeds (pumpkin, sunflower, hemp, chia), mushrooms (porcini, shiitake, button, chestnut), grains (quinoa, oats, buckwheat)*

Iodine helps the body synthesise thyroid hormones, which play an important role in metabolism and the energy production cycle, as well as improving cognitive clarity and focus.

▶ *fish (salmon, mackerel, tuna, cod), shellfish (prawns, mussels, oysters, clams), seaweed (kelp, nori, wakame), dairy products, eggs*

Animal protein is a far richer source of iron than plant protein, so if you're avoiding it during fasting plans, try an iron supplement combined with vitamin C, which will help improve absorption.

Seaweed snacks are top of the class when it comes to iodine. The vitamins, the minerals, the sirtuin-stimulation... you name it. They also make a great snack during 700-calorie days.

3 stop, breathe and get happy:
de-stress and rebalance

Our problem these days is that life is constantly on the go. And it's busy. Work, kids, constantly pinging phones, never being able to switch off because we are too contactable. Most of us are stressed and we think it's normal. It's just the modern world, we tell ourselves.

Stress is real. It's not something you're making up. It's a biochemical reaction that happens in the body, triggering the release of stress hormones that are designed to make you hyper-alert as if you're going to be attacked by a lion. This is the fight-or-flight self-protection method the body and brain use as an immediate response to a perceived threat, but it can be exhausting and miserable when it goes on and on.

GP *tip*

Use the 4-7-8 breathing technique (see page 105) any time you feel stressed. You can do it anywhere – on the school run (like me), in a meeting (also like me) or just before bed to help you wind down for the night.

However, like stress, happiness is also stimulated by a series of chemical reactions. Our brains contain several neurotransmitters – serotonin, oxytocin, endorphins, dopamine and GABA – which give us feelings of joy, relaxation and happiness when they are released.

We are actually predetermined to want to experience pleasure and do everything we can to swerve pain or unhappiness, and these chemicals help us do just that. Happiness is a physical experience, therefore it makes sense to optimise the levels of these neurotransmitters in the body. And apart from reducing stress, this will inevitably impact other aspects of your life, from sleeping better, to improving energy levels, and maintaining a healthy, stable weight. There are several ways to do this – and one of them is through diet.

Remember the principles of hedonic adaptation. Set your own baseline for what makes you happy. This is the key to finding balance for yourself and in everyday life.

GP *tip*

Keeping your hippocampus fired up by memorising something is a great de-stressor. It has been scientifically proven to strengthen cognitive function, helps keep the memory sharp and will make a surprising turn at dinner parties (watch their faces as you recite the first chapter of Anna Karenina after the starter).

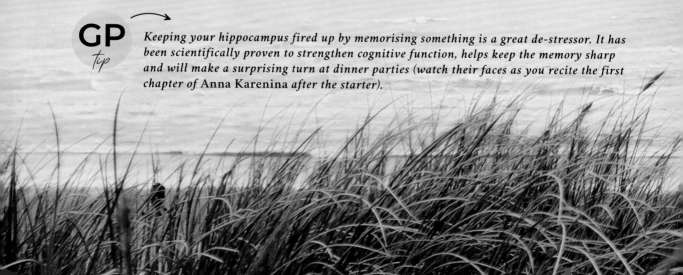

breathe stress away

Periods of stress impact the way we breathe, typically making breaths shallower and therefore reducing oxygen levels. Cells use oxygen to generate energy for every area of the body, so to say that it's essential to life is an understatement. The way – and amount – that we breathe will directly impact our cognitive clarity, energy levels and heart rate. Controlling our breathing is one of the most immediately accessible things we can do to decrease anxiety – and yet we rarely think to use it.

The physical response to stress is meant to be a short-term emergency reaction, but the problem is, it doesn't always get automatically deactivated, meaning the body produces a constant stream of stress hormones. Not only does this lead to endless feelings of anxiety and worry, but it can affect everything from quality of sleep and energy levels, to hormone balance, mental health, nutritional deficiencies and weight gain. Collectively, all these effects will negatively impact how the body ages.

▸ *Breathe in for the count of four, hold for seven counts, then breathe out for eight. This technique slows down the heart rate and signals the brain to override the sympathetic nervous system's fight-or-flight reaction. Give it a few rounds – preferably for no less than five minutes – to experience the full effects.*

adapting to stress with adaptogens

Adaptogens are powerful plants and mushrooms that help maintain homeostasis within the body by increasing its resistance to stress. The by-product of this is that they naturally assist in reducing fatigue by boosting cellular energy and increasing alertness.

▸ **Mushrooms**: *Cordyceps, lion's mane, reishi, maitake, shiitake, chaga*

▸ **Herbs:** *ashwagandha, rhodiola, Siberian ginseng, schisandra, liquorice root, holy basil*

The rule of thumb with adaptogens is the more the merrier, as they all come with slightly different benefits. Mix your favourite adaptogen food sources and look for supplements that combine a few varieties.

boost your 'happy' neurotransmitters

Your brain naturally produces neurotransmitters designed to elevate your mood but they sometimes need a helping hand. The nutrient L-theanine induces calm by stimulating serotonin and GABA, two neurotransmitters that soothe anxiety and increase happiness. Tryptophan, as well as supporting healthy sleep, is another precursor of serotonin and helps the body relax and feel good, while exercise is another way to flood the body with dopamine and endorphins. Oxytocin is known as the 'love hormone'. It can be released by something as simple as hugging a friend or stroking a dog – so don't hold back.

▸ **L-theanine:** *tea leaves, particularly green tea*

▸ **GABA:** *cruciferous vegetables (broccoli, kale, Brussels sprouts, cauliflower), peas, brown rice, mushrooms, sprouted grains, fermented foods (kombucha, kefir, kimchi, miso)*

If you're avoiding caffeine, support your L-theanine intake with supplements.

be kind to yourself

Happiness is not about being perfect. Making mistakes or poor choices, getting things wrong and even behaving badly are all parts of being human. Without these kinds of experiences, we would never evolve. No one gets everything right all the time, and wisdom doesn't come from having led an immaculate life. It comes with letting go of all the things you can't control and finding peace in acceptance.

There will always be people who have more – who are more beautiful, have better relationships, bigger houses, better jobs, shinier cars and thinner waists. You miss out on your life when you spend the whole time chasing things you think you need to make yourself happy. It has been scientifically proven that people who are grateful for what they have live longer and more content lives, so it's worth taking time out to acknowledge the things that are working in your life.

▸ *We are designed to have a spectrum of emotions. The highs are made better in life because of the lows. Let's embrace all of them.*

▸ *Comparing yourself to someone else or being judgemental is ultimately a reflection of how you feel about yourself. After all, we never really know what's going on in the inner corridors of other people's minds and relationships.*

 Perfect is boring. Not one person on the planet hasn't got things wrong in their life (apart from me, my husband would say).

disconnect *to* reconnect

Being constantly contactable doesn't mean we should make ourselves constantly available. We live in a hyper-connected world, where the lines between work and home have dissolved. It is our choice to determine our boundaries between our work and home life and there are a few things we can do to help with that.

▸ *Don't look at your work emails out of working hours, at weekends or on holiday. Make your time off count so you can be present in each area of your life.*

▸ *Note how much time you spend on social media. Settings on your phone will tell you and sometimes the results come as a real surprise. Yes, those videos of dachshunds dressed as firemen are completely charming, but maybe not for two hours.*

▸ *Don't double-screen. It's TV or phone. Not both. You have only one set of eyes and they have to look in the same direction. Pick one or the other!*

▸ *Do you really need devices at the table? We're all guilty of it, but it's a shame to see people staring at their phones and not each other in a restaurant, or children demanding a device to keep them entertained.*

GP *tip* *For young children, make up a little bag of simple craft activities they can do in a restaurant, like colouring and drawing. Then sit back for a relaxing two-hour lunch while they draw incomprehensible pictures of dinosaurs that you have to keep saying are brilliant.*

GP
tip

Social media can be great for staying in touch with people, but nothing beats spending time with friends who make you laugh in real life. Like the ones in front of you. In the room. Just look up from your phone for two minutes. At the ones you invited over.

go green

Sometimes you just have to stop and get out of the house. Studies have proved that spending time in nature can significantly improve your mood, as well as your general health. The idea that the medicinal power of fresh air will help solve problems or provide a much-needed break is not a new one, and for good reason. In our sedentary life, where we are so dominated by technology, the simple act of being outside – moving, breathing and taking in your surroundings – is an easy way to feel restored.

▸ **Spend time outdoors in a green space** – *whether it's a park in a city, a field in the country or a back garden. Scientific research shows that the human eye responds very strongly to the wavelengths emitted by the colour green, which has a calming effect on the nervous system.*

GP
tip

If you don't have a garden, bring the garden to you. Try a window box or houseplants at home or at work. The more the merrier – plus the extra oxygen will help lift your mood and sharpen your focus.

4 get stronger, live longer:
the love affair between exercise and longevity

A lot of research has been done into the relationship between exercise and longevity; along with fasting, it's the most effective method of improving how the body ages. But with so many options to choose from, the world of exercise can become a little bit confusing. How often? What type? Running or walking? Stretching or strengthening?

The answer is: a bit of everything. All movement is good. Exercise not only helps build muscle, but also has a cellular effect on the body. It activates sirtuins, the longevity genes, and helps the body flush out senescent cells – dysfunctional, redundant cells that can cause multiple health issues. Evacuate the building, please!

Getting active is not only incredibly powerful for longevity, it's essential for boosting energy levels, improving sleep, reducing inflammation, maintaining a balanced weight and improving mental health. Exercise is also incredibly rewarding. Its effects on the body and mind are often immediate – no one goes for a brisk, energising walk and comes home thinking, 'Ugh, that was horrible, what a mistake.' So stop reading this, get up and go out. Chop, chop, shake a leg.

GP *tip*

Calling all those with sedentary jobs – try a standing desk. Or get up and walk around when you're making a call. If you're standing in a queue, go up and down on your toes like a policeman (don't get overexcited and arrest someone; that is not allowed).

daily low-impact movement

Don't underestimate the impact of small, constant movement – like taking the dog for a walk or hoovering your home. This all contributes to your daily step count, one of the simplest gateways into low-impact exercise, and helps to start the process of hormesis and autophagy.

▶ *The daily recommended step count is 7,000–10,000. In one go, 10,000 steps would roughly equate to just over an hour's walk – but moving throughout the day contributes* to that target, which means it's more likely that a 30–45 minute brisk walk will help you reach the 10k goal. Unless you are having a duvet/Netflix day (at least reach for the remote a few times to flex your triceps; work with me here).

▶ *Get moving. Choose walking over other forms of transport. Use the stairs instead of escalators. Get off the bus or tube stop earlier and walk the rest of the way. Cycle to work or just for fun. Even a walk around the block after work will help to bring a sense of closure for the day, especially when so many of us are now working from home.*

Try touching your toes. Was it easy or was it hell? Don't underestimate the importance of stretching. Maintaining flexibility through yoga or stretching at home helps strengthen and lengthen the muscles, protecting the joints and improving posture.

 If you're curious to know your step count, download a pedometer app or use a smartwatch to track your steps. Slightly easier than counting them yourself.

cardio

Cardio or aerobic exercise involves any kind |of rhythmical movement that gets your blood pumping, lungs working and heart rate going (watching *Bridgerton* doesn't count). This means being out of breath (entering a state of hypoxia). Lowering oxygen levels stimulates a mitochondrial hormetic response, which has been shown to increase insulin sensitivity and balance blood sugar levels. The calorie-burning helps achieve or maintain a healthy weight as well as building muscle, while the activation of sirtuin genes and inflammation reduction improves the ageing process.

▶ *Upgrade your daily step count with running or brisk walking (no dawdling – walk as if you think you left the iron on and need to get home) for 30 minutes, five days a week.*

▶ *If your target is to lose weight and improve fitness levels, increase your daily activity depending on your general health and goals.*

▶ *When it comes to cardio, the world is your oyster – hiking, cycling, swimming, rowing, skipping, boxing, trampolining – do anything that involves dynamic movement where you lose your breath.*

 Vary the intensity and length of daily physical exercise. It's easy to move from short-term stress on the body to long term by doing too much. Balance, balance, balance.

 Try organised sport. Force your children to play tennis, football or rounders with you to get them off the sofa and reduce your chances of having boozy weekends and falling asleep in the middle of the afternoon.

 Run up and down stairs. Sounds horrendous (it sort of is), but it's really easy, involves no prep or having to get changed and will get you into a mild state of hypoxia.

 The way to tell if you're hypoxic is if you can't easily hold a conversation. Go hiking with someone you don't really like and get fit quicker! Yay!

Yes, we all want abs you could break a plank of wood against – but it's important to strengthen all muscle groups, so ensure that you do a variety of muscle-building exercises.

build your muscles

Strength is important. Muscles are built when they are challenged. The greater our muscle mass, the more calories we burn, and the better and more efficiently our bodies function. This is where high intensity training comes in. It activates hormone-sensitive lipase, the enzyme that mobilises and burns fat. All this and it charges up the process of autophagy – a winning combination of hormetic stressors to reduce weight and live for eternity!

▶ *Choose resistance training that uses the contraction of the muscles to build strength, such as HiiT, spinning, Pilates Reformer or gym programmes that use resistance bands, medicine balls, dumbbells or weights.*

▶ *Research recommends at least 70–80 minutes of strength training in total a week – ideally short bursts spread over a few days.*

Resistance training is more beneficial when your body has time to recover and build on the effort you put in. Doing too much can lead to cortisol spikes, so try not to train on consecutive days.

Keep ankle or wrist weights handy – leave them by the door and put them on before walking the dog, picking the kids up from school or going out for a martini (you've earned it).

As little as 15 minutes of resistance training is enough for one session, and you don't necessarily need to go to the gym. Try push-ups, sit-ups or lunges in the privacy of your home or, indeed, in front of your boss (pay rise guaranteed?).

Get involved with protein bars as a healthy and convenient snack when training. They're great quality these days and there are many vegan varieties available. Make sure you choose them over energy bars, which tend to be high in sugar.

5 clean up: *send unwanted chemicals packing*

The liver is one of the hardest-working organs in the body. It stores glycogen (converted glucose) to help balance blood sugar levels, assists in the breakdown of fats and transportation of fatty acids and hormones, and acts as a chemical filter to process anything our bodies don't need. That means everything from redundant hormones that no longer serve us, to the alcohol we drink, pollution we inadvertently inhale and chemicals we put in, on or around our bodies – perfume, washing powder, cosmetics, pesticides in food, cleaning products. You name it, the liver will have to deal with it. 'Busy' doesn't do justice to the hours this organ puts in for us.

So it stands to reason that a healthy, robust liver will assist all the work the body needs to do to ensure homeostasis. It will affect everything from the way we sleep and how energised we feel, to our hormone balance, the state of our immune system and our inflammation levels. It supports the role of autophagy in cleansing the body, while benefitting from the recharging effects this process has.

It goes without saying that most of us live in a world where chemicals are just a part of life, so don't panic if you're not living in the Swiss mountains or in an oxygen tank. It will help, however, to be aware of how to minimise exposure in our homes and from our lifestyle, when possible, to improve in any way we can the chemical balance within the body.

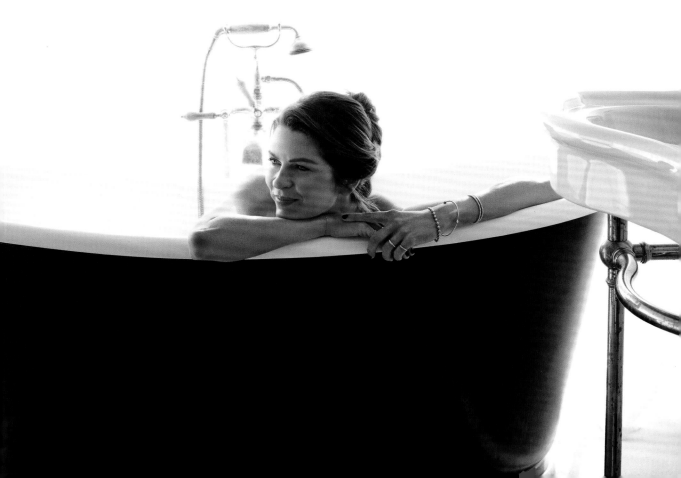

take a closer look at home...

Many of us introduce unnecessary chemicals into our homes in ways of which we might not be aware, and our livers will have to process all of them. From plastic bottles, food containers and food wrap, to cleaning products, washing detergents and chemically-enhanced nonstick kitchenware, they sneak in everywhere.

► Replace plastic kitchenware with glass or stainless steel bottles and jars, silicone lids and pouches and beeswax wraps.

► Swap chemical washing detergents and cleaning products with eco-friendly, organic equivalents.

► Replace old or scratched nonstick pans with stainless steel, enamel, ceramic or cast iron alternatives.

 Food heated in plastic containers will absorb harmful chemicals. Always transfer food to an oven-safe glass or ceramic dish before heating.

 Plastic bottles are not only bad for the environment, they are particularly harmful in hot weather, seeping their evil chemicals into the liquid they contain. Always try to stick to reusable BPA-free bottles, where possible. Good for you, good for the planet.

 Get mixing your own toxin-free cleaning solutions. One part vinegar to one part water is great on glass and stainless steel; add a dash of bicarbonate of soda for tougher stains.

skin solutions

Many popular products contain chemicals, but again, it's not a case of removing everything you love from your skincare routine or make-up bag. Instead, it's worth trying to find a balance between your favourite products and reducing your chemical intake where possible.

► Keep an eye out for listed ingredients. Parabens, sulphates, artificial fragrance and phthalates, are among the worst culprits.

► Choose mineral sunscreens, which sit on the skin without being absorbed like their chemical-based counterparts.

► Foaming skincare products indicate chemicals – replace with products that use more natural ingredients.

► Synthetic antiperspirants are packed with chemicals and parabens, which get into the body's system and can disrupt hormone levels. Swap them for natural-based deodorants that allow the skin to breathe.

► Mainstream brand cosmetics and fragrances tend to contain a lot of artificial ingredients, so try to use them for only special occasions and look at organic-based products for day-to-day use.

GP *tip*

And now for a little beauty trick. Opt for natural products on your body's larger surface area and your favourite chemical products on the smaller surface area of your face.

GP *tip*

Reduce the chemical intake of your favourite perfume by spraying it onto your clothes rather than your skin. You'll still smell like a goddess, but with a healthy liver.

GP *tip*

Your mouth is extremely porous, so instead of swallowing down a ton of chemicals, switch off-the-shelf toothpaste with an organic variety.

GP *tip*

If you're wedded to your favourite haircare brand, try washing your hair upside down in the shower – step out of the water and stick your head under it, instead of letting the product wash over your body as you rinse. Cunning.

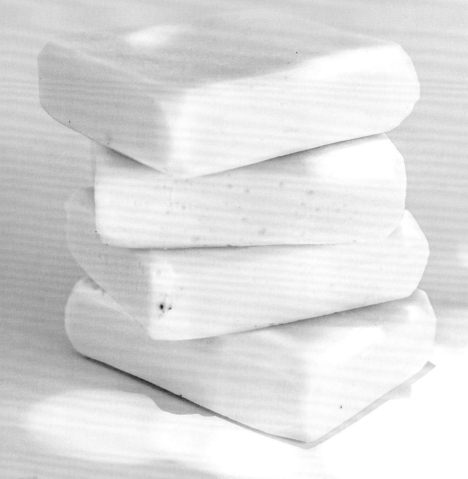

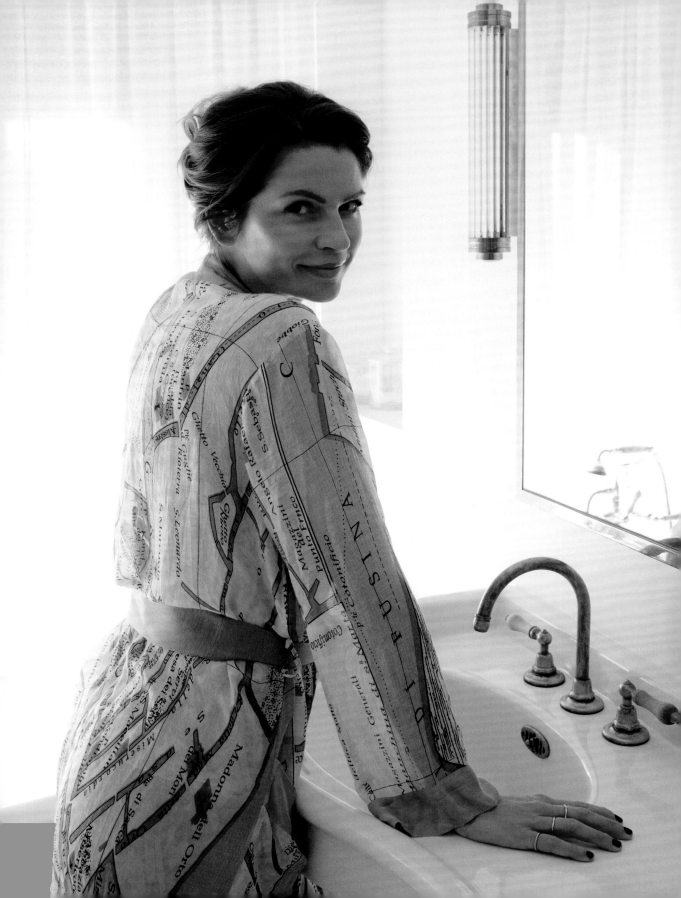

When it comes to meat and fish, better quality, less often is preferred. Choose sparingly, but choose well.

liver-loving menus

How to strike a balance between organic and non-organic? There's no question that organic products are healthier and better for the planet – but they're expensive and don't always last. What can help is to instead make smart choices about when to go organic, if always choosing organic is not an option.

▶ **Animal products:** *apart from the fact they are reared far more humanely, organic meat, fish, eggs and dairy do not contain the hormones and antibiotics that are typically used on non-organic equivalents. It's worth prioritising this category for organic options because of how the chemicals will have been ingested by the animal.*

▶ **Fruit and vegetables:** *chemical fertilisers are commonly used on mass-produced fruit and vegetables, but if the chemically-sprayed skin is always removed, as you do for an avocado or an orange, then non-organic is acceptable.*

Remove pesticides with a special fruit and vegetable brush (you can even get a cleaning solution to go with it). Give them a good scrub in water so that you keep the nutrient-rich skin but remove the bad stuff.

Remove pesticides with a special fruit and vegetable brush (you can even get a cleaning solution to go with it). Give them a good scrub in water so that you keep the nutrient-rich skin but remove the bad stuff.

Seasonal fruit and vegetable boxes and organic meat deliveries are not only a great way to support small businesses, but they help reduce the carbon footprint from buying ingredients from across the world. Take a look at what's on offer in your area.

Embrace the cold. Organic soft fruit can be expensive, so buying it frozen is a good alternative. It's still full of fantastic nutrients and lasts a lot longer in the freezer.

6 stars of the supplement world: *taking things to the next level*

Think of supplements as a major support network. Taken in conjunction with a healthy diet, these concentrated nutrients can make major biochemical improvements within the body. I am very keen on supplements and regularly prescribe them to my clients alongside providing dietary advice, as nutrient deficiencies are common. Unfortunately, the realities of everyday life, from stress and poor sleep, to alcohol and pollution exposure, mean our bodies are under constant assault from all angles, draining our nutrient resources as they're redirected to depleted areas. Supplements underpin all the good work of a healthy diet and lifestyle, ensuring that nutrient levels are topped up. I couldn't love them more.

In this section, I include my must-haves for everyday health, plus boosters for specific goals and longevity supplements. I encourage you to try a few and see which ones you like. They are all backed by scientific research, so find the ones that work for you and the way you live life.

a little note on supplement shopping

▶ **POTENCY:** compare the dosage on the labels of trusted brands. The higher the nutrient content, the more significant the effects on your body.

▶ **BIOAVAILABILITY:** good brands will offer nutrients that are more easily absorbed by the body, often combining them to maximise their impact.

▶ **CONVENIENCE:** choose tablets, capsules, powder or drinks – whatever you feel will encourage you to keep taking them.

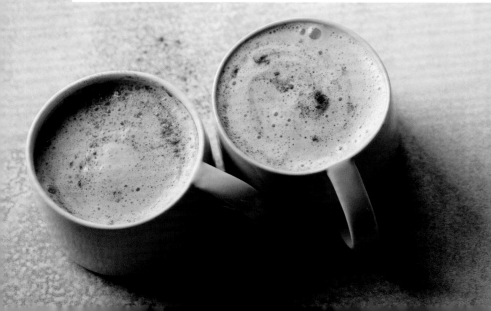

a good-quality multi-nutrient
(containing all essential vitamins and minerals)

Having a baseline for all-round support is a great foundation for general health. Each system within the body will affect another – for example, poor sleep leads to decreased energy, slow cognitive function, weight gain or a sluggish immune system. Being deficient in a nutrient will eventually initiate a cascade effect, where different areas begin to be impacted by one low-functioning trigger.

IF weight loss support

▸ **PROBIOTICS:** help to balance the intestinal microbiota, which assists with healthy weight loss and appetite control among many other benefits

▸ **B VITAMINS:** essential for restoring energy levels by ensuring the body uses glucose as energy, rather than storing it as triglycerides in adipose tissue

▸ **GLUCOMANNAN:** a plant-sourced soluble fibre that attracts water and forms a gel-like substance in the stomach, balancing blood sugar levels and feelings of satiety, while also feeding healthy bacteria in the intestine

▸ **GREEN TEA EXTRACT:** rich in antioxidants and phytochemicals, it reduces inflammation, supports the immune system and helps break down and release stored fat in adipose tissue.

▸ **CHROMIUM:** a mineral that increases insulin efficiency as it transports glucose to the cells for energy, balancing blood sugar levels and reducing cravings.

a little note on apple cider vinegar

Welcome to the many talents of apple cider vinegar. It helps balance blood sugar levels and improves insulin sensitivity, both of which contribute to healthy weight loss. It also supports liver function and digestive health by normalising stomach pH and promoting healthy microflora. Apple cider vinegar all day, every day.

GP *tip*

Try this apple cider vinegar liver-supporting, longevity-loving, energising mega mix: 1 tablespoon apple cider vinegar, 1 tablespoon lemon juice, ¼ teaspoon ground turmeric, 200ml (7fl oz) warm water, a squeeze of agave syrup and a pinch of cayenne pepper. Mix up and drink up first thing in the morning on an empty stomach.

IMMUNITY AND ANTI-INFLAMMATION

- Turmeric
- Omega 3
- Vitamin D
- Resveratrol
- Quercetin
- Zinc
- Selenium
- Vitamin C
- Probiotics
- Medicinal mushrooms (*reishi, maitake, shiitake, Cordyceps, lion's mane*)

LIVER SUPPORT AND CLEANSING

- Omega 3
- Probiotics
- Turmeric
- Curcumin
- Green superfood powders (*wheatgrass, spirulina, chlorella, broccoli, kale*)
- L-methionine
- Green tea extract
- ALA
- Selenium
- Choline

SLEEP AND RELAXATION

- Magnesium
- 5-HTP
- L-theanine
- Omega 3
- Adaptogens (*rhodiola, ashwagandha, Siberian ginseng*)
- L-glycine
- Vitamin D

DIGESTION AND ABSORPTION

- Antimicrobials (*grapefruit seed extract, oregano, berberine*)
- L-glutamine
- Digestive enzyme complex (*including HCL*)
- Probiotics
- Slippery elm
- Curcumin
- Wheatgrass

COGNITIVE AND EMOTIONAL WELL-BEING

- 5-HTP
- L-theanine
- GABA
- Probiotics
- Adaptogens
- Omega 3
- Vitamin B complex

ENERGY AND VITALITY

- Vitamin B complex
- Red, purple and blue superfood powders (*acai, goji, bilberry, blueberry, blackberry, cherry*)
- Iron
- Iodine
- Adaptogens (*rhodiola, ashwagandha, Siberian ginseng*)
- CoQ10
- Green tea extract
- Magnesium

FOR DE-STRESSING AND REBALANCING

- Adaptogens (*rhodiola, ashwagandha, Siberian ginseng*)
- Magnesium
- Probiotics
- Vitamin B complex
- Vitamin D
- Glucomannan

and now... hands up if you remember NAD+?

Anyone? The battery chargers of the cell? The ones that fire up mitochondria within the cell? Help repair DNA? The ones that we would fall down and die without because that's how important they are? The ones that deplete as we age? Yes, those ones. They're the key to healthy longevity as you're about to discover…

For boosting longevity

All the supplements mentioned opposite will naturally support improved longevity, but research is also revealing nutrients that target specific longevity pathways in the body, activating sirtuin genes.

We're in relatively early days, but it's an incredibly exciting and progressive area of scientific study that is continuing to deliver fascinating results.

- ▶ **Quercetin:** this antioxidant flavonoid improves NAD+ levels, reduces inflammation, activates SIRT longevity genes and assists in clearing senescent cells (*see page 19*).

- ▶ **NMN** (nicotinamide mononucleotide) **and NR** (nicotinamide riboside): these are biological precursors to NAD+, as NAD+ itself cannot be supplemented on its own. Research has suggested NMN and NR may boost energy, increase insulin sensitivity, lower inflammation and support genome stability by repairing DNA and boosting mitochondria. Some studies are even exploring whether they imitate the effects of calorie restriction, potentially supporting positive changes in body composition, like healthy weight loss.

- ▶ **Resveratrol:** a powerful polyphenol, it activates sirtuin genes, reduces inflammation and oxidative stress, increases mitochondrial activity, boosts the metabolism, helps balance blood sugar levels and supports healthy cognitive function.

- ▶ **Spermidine:** known to stimulate autophagy, it plays a crucial role in apoptosis, preserving DNA, lipid metabolism and both the function and the survival of the cell.

- ▶ **Medicinal mushrooms** (reishi, shiitake, maitake, lion's mane, chaga, cordyceps): all containing the compound beta-glucan (a prebiotic that feeds intestinal bacteria), these adaptogens are powerful anti-inflammatories, reduce oxidative damage and help support the immune system.

- ▶ **Astaxanthin:** an antioxidant carotenoid found in red algae, it upregulates autophagy, is a strong anti-inflammatory, preserves neuron integrity, reduces oxidative stress and helps support mitochondrial function.

- ▶ **Berberine:** a bioactive compound found in plants, it helps balance blood sugar levels and insulin sensitivity, supporting healthy weight loss. It has antimicrobial properties that improve intestinal microflora and reduce premature cellular senescence. Known to stimulate mitohormesis, it increases mitochondrial function and energy levels.

GP golden rules for longevity

the GP principles for a longevity diet

1 **PROTEIN IS EVERYTHING:** always include a variety of protein sources.

2 **THE COMPLEX WORLD OF CARBOHYDRATES:** choose the colourful, high-fibre, non-starchy kind.

3 **FUN FACTS ABOUT FATS:** maintain a healthy balance with focus on essential fatty acids.

4 **FANTASTIC LONGEVITY-LOVING FOODS:** increase intake of sirtuin-stimulating, anti-inflammatory, digestion-supporting foods.

5 **DRINK UP:** keep fluid levels topped up regularly throughout the day.

GP longevity IF plans

▶ **SUPER-CHARGE 700**
▶ **RESET 700**
▶ **LIVE LONG 16:8**

longevity triggers

1. **RELEASE THE SHOCK PROTEINS!** Expose yourself regularly to hot and cold therapy.
2. **TIME FOR BED:** helping yourself sleep better will naturally increase energy levels and vice versa.
3. **STOP, BREATHE AND GET HAPPY:** de-stress physically and mentally and focus on what brings you joy.
4. **GET STRONGER, LIVE LONGER:** exercise regularly with a blend of resistance training, muscle-stretching and cardio-boosting physical activity.
5. **CLEAN UP:** support liver function by reducing the amount of chemical exposure in your home and what you eat.
6. **THE MAGIC OF SUPPLEMENTS:** boost the body through IF plans and everyday life with targeted longevity nutrients.

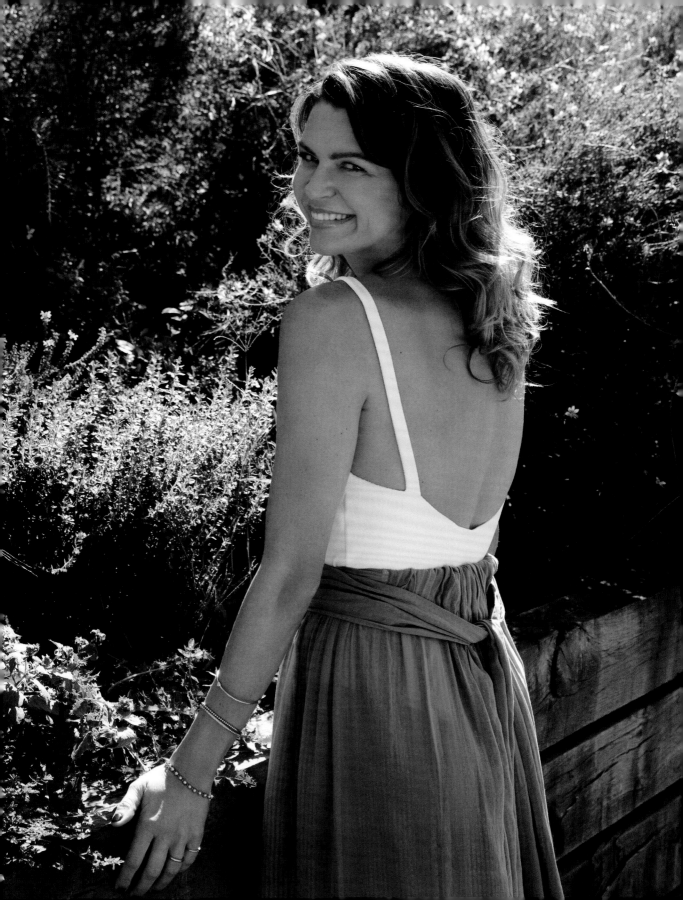

the recipes

Welcome to the recipe section, with lots of delicious ideas to get you inspired, and to fit the longevity plans. Easy to follow (honestly, who has the patience?) and packed with plenty of super nutrients, I've included lots of variety to ensure there's something for everyone. I can't wait for you to find your favourites...

700 day recipes

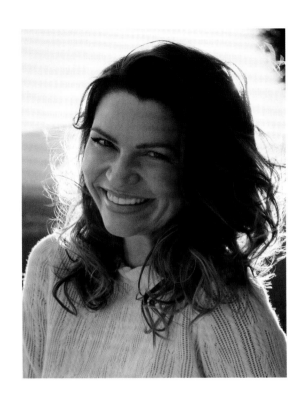
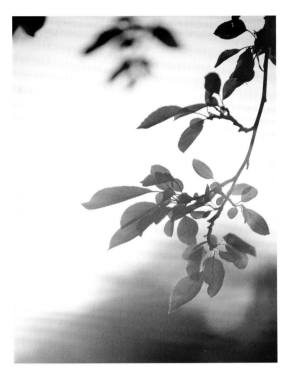
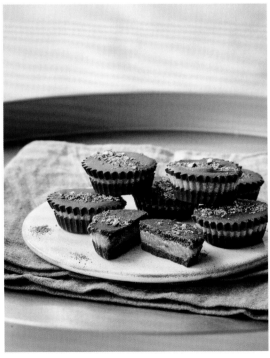
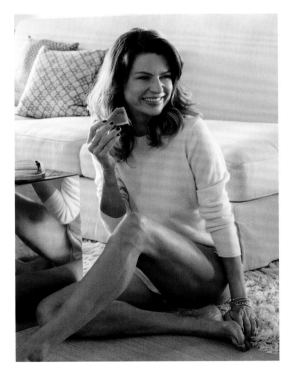

if using vegetarian
Parmesan-style or
vegan cheese

gluten
free   veggie

700 day

mini breakfast frittatas

serves 4

olive oil, for greasing
6 organic or free-range eggs
2 carrots, grated
1 red pepper, cored, deseeded
   and chopped
large handful of kale (20g/¾oz),
   stalks removed and chopped,
   or 30g/1oz spinach, roughly
   chopped
2 shallots, finely chopped
2 garlic cloves, grated
8 basil leaves, torn
¼ teaspoon ground cumin
¼ teaspoon cayenne pepper
30g (1oz) Parmesan cheese or
   vegetarian/vegan alternative,
   finely grated
sea salt and freshly ground
   pepper

A cute, colourful, super-low-calorie start to the day – welcome to mini breakfast frittatas, which incorporate lots of longevity-supporting phytochemicals (plant pigments). For those skipping breakfast as part of 16:8, don't feel left out. These little guys are extremely versatile – you can throw in literally whatever vegetables you have in the refrigerator. They make a delicious breakfast, but I love them as a cold snack, great to bring to work. I quite want one now, actually...

Preheat the oven to 210°C (410°F), Gas Mark 6½ and grease a 6-hole muffin tin using a little olive oil.

Crack the eggs into a bowl and beat, before adding all the other ingredients – the carrots, pepper, kale, shallots, garlic, basil, cumin, cayenne pepper, Parmesan, salt and pepper. The mixture should be roughly half egg, half vegetables.

Spoon the mixture evenly into the greased muffin tin and bake for about 15 minutes. They should be set in the centre, so give the tin a little jiggle to check.

Remove from the oven and let them cool a little before serving.

super-low
cal

PREP 15 minutes	COOK 15 minutes	CALORIES 157

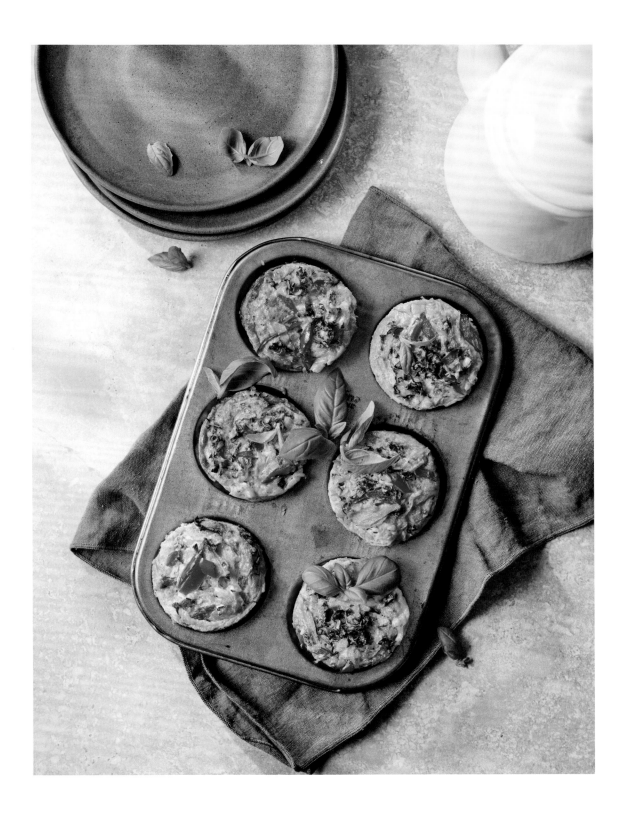

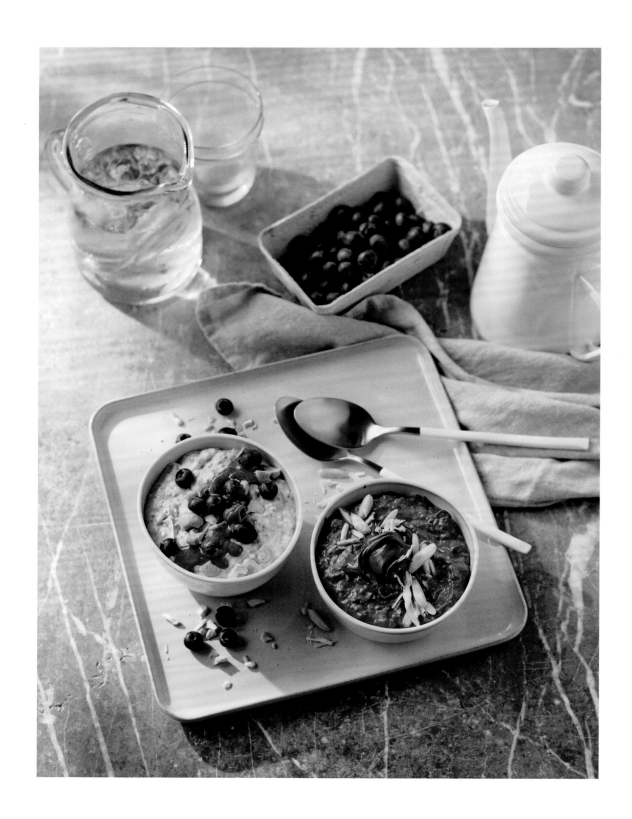

if using gluten-free certified oats and oat milk

gluten free	dairy free	vegan

700 day

vegan overnight oats

serves 2

base recipe
45g (1½oz) rolled oats (gluten-free, if preferred)

120g (4¼oz) coconut or nut yogurt (e.g. almond)

3 tablespoons vegan protein powder

120ml (4fl oz) oat, coconut or nut milk (e.g. almond)

1 tablespoon agave syrup

blueberry, flaxseed & cashew nut
1 quantity Base Recipe

½ tablespoon flaxseeds

20g (¾oz) cashew nuts, chopped

100g (3½oz) blueberries

1 tablespoon almond butter

chocolate almond
1 quantity Base Recipe

1 tablespoon raw cacao powder

1 tablespoon chopped almonds

1 tablespoon dairy-free vegan-friendly organic chocolate and hazelnut spread

super-low cal

This is where breakfast gets creative. The oat mixture acts as the base, with an additional protein powder boost to keep blood sugar levels nice and steady. The good thing about this recipe is that you can decide what to add to the oats depending on where your mood takes you. I've included some of my favourite suggestions to get the ball rolling. For breakfast dodgers, this could also be an afternoon snack. I will fight anyone who says it can't.

Prepare the base oat mixture by adding all the ingredients to a container with a lid and mix well.

blueberry, flaxseed & cashew nut overnight oats

Prepare the base oat mixture as above. Stir in the flaxseeds and cashew nuts (keep a few over for serving), cover and leave in the refrigerator overnight.

Serve the next day with the reserved chopped cashew nuts, the blueberries and almond butter on top.

chocolate almond overnight oats

Prepare the base oat mixture as above. Stir in the cacao powder and chopped almonds (reserve a few for serving), cover and leave in the refrigerator overnight.

Serve the next day with the reserved almonds and a dollop of vegan chocolate and hazelnut spread.

PREP 10 minutes	CHILL overnight	CALORIES 259 for base recipe with oat milk 395 for blueberry flavour 377 for chocolate flavour

gluten
free

dairy
free

veggie

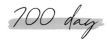

100 day

mediterranean baked eggs

serves 2

1 tablespoon olive oil
1 courgette, grated
1 garlic clove, grated
1 teaspoon chilli flakes
400g (14oz) can of chopped
  tomatoes
80g (3oz) kale, stalks removed
  and roughly chopped
4 organic or free-range eggs
6 cherry tomatoes, halved
sea salt and freshly ground
  pepper

to serve

30g (1oz) parsley, chopped
30g (1oz) basil leaves
1 red chilli, deseeded and sliced

The Mediterranean diet has a vast array of vegetables and plenty of good fats like olive oil, all of which contribute to long and healthy lives. This dish comes with the added bonus of phytonutrients from the vegetables, all of which contribute to healthy longevity. Throw in any herbs you like – I use basil and parsley, but a few snips of chives over the top would be delicious, too.

Preheat the oven to 200°C (400°F), Gas Mark 6.

Heat a frying pan (with a lid) over a medium heat. Add the oil and courgette and fry for 3 minutes, stirring regularly. Then add the garlic, chilli flakes and canned tomatoes and cook for a further 8 minutes.

Add the kale and mix it into the tomato sauce and season well. Then make four little wells in the sauce and crack an egg into each one. Place the cherry tomatoes around the eggs and cover with the lid. Cook for 4–5 minutes or until the whites are set and the yolks are still runny (cook for slightly longer if you prefer them firmer).

Serve with the parsley, basil and sliced chilli.

super-low
cal

PREP 10 minutes	COOK 20 minutes	CALORIES 270

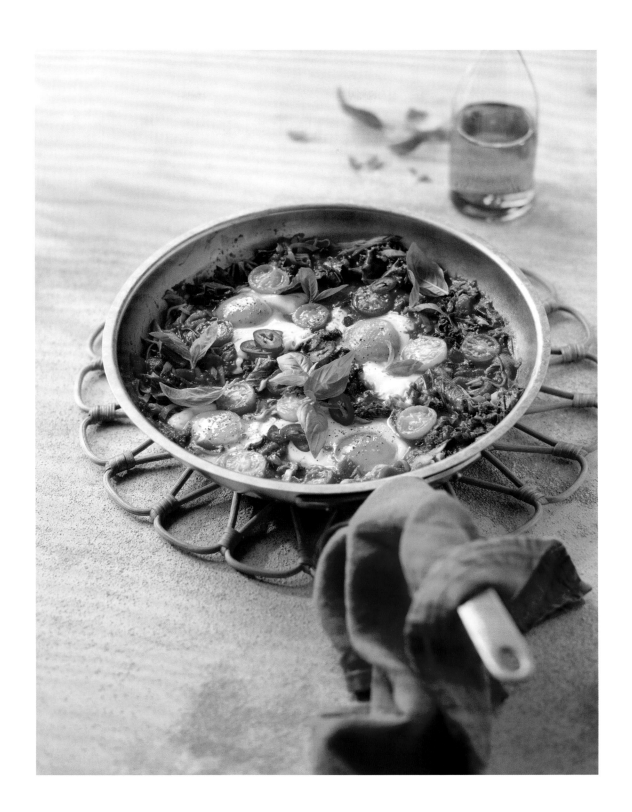

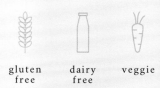

gluten free   dairy free   veggie

100 day

cinnamon buckwheat pancakes

makes 15 pancakes

1 tablespoon coconut oil
150ml (5fl oz) unsweetened oat
  milk, at room temperature
½ teaspoon apple cider vinegar
110g (4oz) buckwheat flour
½ teaspoon bicarbonate of soda
1 organic or free-range egg, at
  room temperature
1 tablespoon agave syrup
2 teaspoons nut butter (cashew,
  almond), to serve (per pancake)
raw cocoa shavings, to serve

Rather misleadingly given its name, buckwheat is not actually wheat. It comes from a seed, is naturally gluten-free and is high in plant protein. The batter will keep in the refrigerator for 2–3 days if you don't want to use it all at once. And when it comes to serving suggestions, the world's your oyster (as long as you keep it super-low cal). I personally love eating them with omega 3-rich nut butter and a sprinkling of raw cocoa shavings, which contain sirtuin-stimulating polyphenols.

Melt the coconut oil in a small pan and then pour into a small heatproof bowl. Set aside to cool. The time it takes you to prepare everything else will probably be enough for this.

Pour the oat milk and apple cider vinegar into a small jug. Add the buckwheat flour and bicarbonate of soda to a bowl.

Add the egg and agave syrup to the coconut oil once it has cooled, then beat together. Add this, along with the oat milk mixture, to the buckwheat flour. Mix well.

Heat a frying pan over a medium heat and add 2 tablespoons of batter per pancake to the pan. You can pour it straight from the jug, but just remember, these pancakes are not huge. When the mixture starts to bubble – usually around a minute or so – flip them over. The second side will take less time, but you're aiming for a light golden colour. Serve with nut butter, or kefir or nut yogurt mixed with some mixed seeds, or a handful of berries.

super-low cal

PREP 8 minutes	COOK 10 minutes	CALORIES 53 per pancake

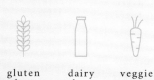

gluten
free

dairy
free

veggie

700 day

gluten-free super seed crackers

makes 48 crackers

100g (3½oz) flaxseeds, plus extra
    to garnish
50g (1¾oz) pumpkin seeds
50g (1¾oz) sunflower seeds
100g (3½oz) mixed nuts
    (almonds, cashew nuts,
    hazelnuts, Brazil nuts, walnuts)
leaves of a small sprig of
    rosemary
1 organic or free-range egg
1 teaspoon garlic powder
½ teaspoon apple cider vinegar
2 tablespoons water
sea salt and freshly ground
    pepper
black sesame seeds, to garnish
    (optional)

For those that love toast, this is a great alternative. Protein-rich and gluten-free, these crunchy little crackers are delicious for breakfast or as a snack. Eat them by themselves or use them as a base on which to spread your favourite dips. All the nuts and seeds in these crackers are like an omega 3 rocket of goodness – your shiny skin and (suddenly?) balanced moods will attest to that.

Preheat the oven to 180°C (350°F), Gas Mark 4 and line two baking trays with nonstick baking paper.

Place the seeds, nuts and rosemary leaves in a blender and blitz until they form fine grains. Tip the mixture into a bowl and add the egg, garlic powder, apple cider vinegar, water and some seasoning, mixing well to form a dough (don't worry if it seems a bit stiff – it's meant to be).

Cut the dough in half, place each half on a separate lined baking tray and roll them into rectangles with a rolling pin – you want them thin, so aim for around 2–3mm (¹⁄₁₆–⅛ inch) thick.

Cut the dough into slices (about 24 per tray), sprinkle them with some water and scatter over the black sesame seeds (if using) and extra flaxseeds. Bake them in the oven for 12–15 minutes and then leave them to cool and crisp up.

They'll keep in a tin, so dip into them throughout the week – particularly if you have some hummus handy.

super-low
cal

PREP 20 minutes	COOK 12–15 minutes	CALORIES 35 per pancake

gluten
free

100 day

chickpea, spinach &
smoked salmon pancakes

serves 2

125g (4½oz) chickpea flour
175ml (6fl oz) warm water
small handful of spinach (approx.
  30g/1oz)
½ tablespoon olive oil
2 slices (40g/1½oz) of smoked
  salmon, torn
30g (1oz) feta, crumbled
squeeze of lemon juice
1 tablespoon chopped chives
sea salt and freshly ground pepper

Pancakes are extremely versatile and don't need to be restricted to just breakfast. This particular recipe involves protein-packed smoked salmon and chickpeas, with some vibrant, iron-rich spinach thrown in for good measure, but feel free to adapt with whatever is handy in the refrigerator. That's the beauty of pancakes – they go with anything.

Add the chickpea flour, water and spinach to a blender, season well and blitz until smooth.

To make each pancake, heat the oil in a smallish frying pan over a medium heat and pour in 3 tablespoons of the batter. Give it a good swirl around the pan until the mixture is nice and thin. Cook for about 1–1½ minutes before flipping it over (a flick of the wrist for the reckless or a spatula for the sensible) to cook on the other side for no more than about 30 seconds. Remove the cooked pancake from the pan and keep warm while you repeat this step to cook the rest of the batter.

Serve topped with the smoked salmon, feta, lemon juice and chives. Take a photo and Instagram it (okay, don't do that).

medium
calorie

PREP 10 minutes	COOK 30 minutes	CALORIES 343

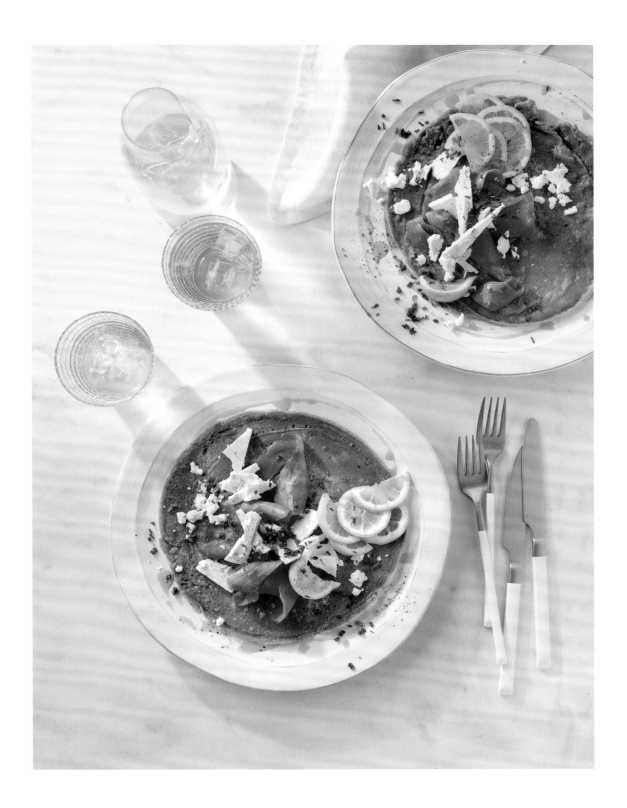

dairy
free

healthy florentine pizza

serves 2

2 wholemeal tortillas
2 tablespoons tomato purée
2 garlic cloves, grated
¼ red onion, thinly sliced
30g (1oz) jarred artichoke hearts
  in brine, chopped
30g (1oz) chestnut mushrooms,
  thinly sliced
2 slices of prosciutto, torn
2 organic or free-range eggs
65g (2¼oz) rocket
sea salt and freshly ground pepper

Look. We all love pizza – but sadly, it isn't allowed for anyone who is fasting. Sad face. But wait! This alternative has an egg on it! And artichokes (you have to get the ones in brine though, not oil, otherwise you might as well just order a takeaway pizza). Seriously, though, the base gets crispy around the edges, the tomato purée is rich in lycopene and there's even prosciutto – the closest you're going to get to pepperoni at this point. You're welcome!

Preheat the oven to 200°C (400°F), Gas Mark 6 and line a large baking tray with foil.

Wrap the tortillas loosely in foil and warm them through in the oven for 5 minutes. You can also heat them in a large, dry frying pan over a medium heat, flipping them after a minute or so, if you prefer. Then place them on the foil-lined tray.

Mix the tomato purée and garlic together in a small bowl and then spread it over the tortillas, like a pizza base. Scatter over the onion, bits of artichoke heart, mushrooms and prosciutto, before breaking an egg into the centre of each tortilla.

Season both and then carefully put them into the oven. Cook until the whites are set and the yolks are still runny – around 10 minutes. The prosciutto should have crisped up a bit at the edges, too. Nice.

Remove from the oven and garnish with the rocket.

medium
calorie

PREP 10 minutes	COOK 15 minutes	CALORIES 306

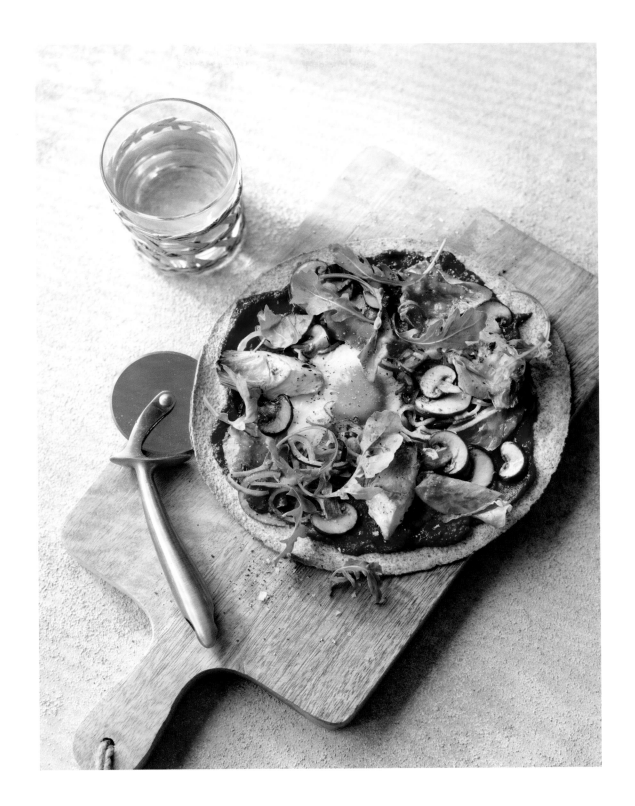

fiery fish tacos

serves 2

for the fish

250g (9oz) white fish fillet (skin-on) of your choice (haddock, cod)
1 teaspoon garlic powder
2 tablespoons smoked paprika
sea salt and freshly ground pepper

for the sauce

100g (3½oz) Greek or live natural yogurt
½ tablespoon chipotle paste or sriracha
juice of ½ lime
sea salt and freshly ground pepper

to serve

4 small wholemeal tortillas, warmed
¼ small red cabbage, finely shredded
1 red chilli or jalapeño, deseeded and sliced
a few fresh coriander leaves

A few little tweaks and everyone's favourite fish tacos are able to make it into the fasting recipe hall of fame. I've made these ones nice and spicy, as this gives the metabolism a healthy boost, while the white fish is obviously a fantastic source of protein, omega 3 and just about anything that's good for you that you can think of. You'll feel your brain getting bigger practically as you eat them.

Preheat the oven to 220°C (425°F), Gas Mark 7 and line a baking tray with foil.

Place the fish on the foil-lined tray and season with the garlic powder, smoked paprika and salt and pepper. How long you cook the fish for in the oven will depend on how thick it is, but 250g (9oz) should typically take around 25–30 minutes. If the fillet is thin, it will take less time – just keep an eye on it.

While the fish is cooking, start on the other elements. For the sauce, mix the yogurt, chipotle paste or sriracha and lime juice in a small bowl and season.

Remove the fish from the oven but leave the oven turned on. Loosely wrap the tortillas in foil and warm them in the oven for 5 minutes. Alternatively, you can warm them in a dry frying pan over a medium heat.

Flake the fish off its skin into nice chunky pieces. Lay out the tortillas and add a portion of the red cabbage, chilli or jalapeño, fish, sauce and coriander to each one. Fold the bottom of each tortilla up, then fold both sides over, leaving the top open. Then shut your eyes and pretend you're on the beach in Mexico.

medium calorie

PREP 15 minutes	COOK 35 minutes	CALORIES 351

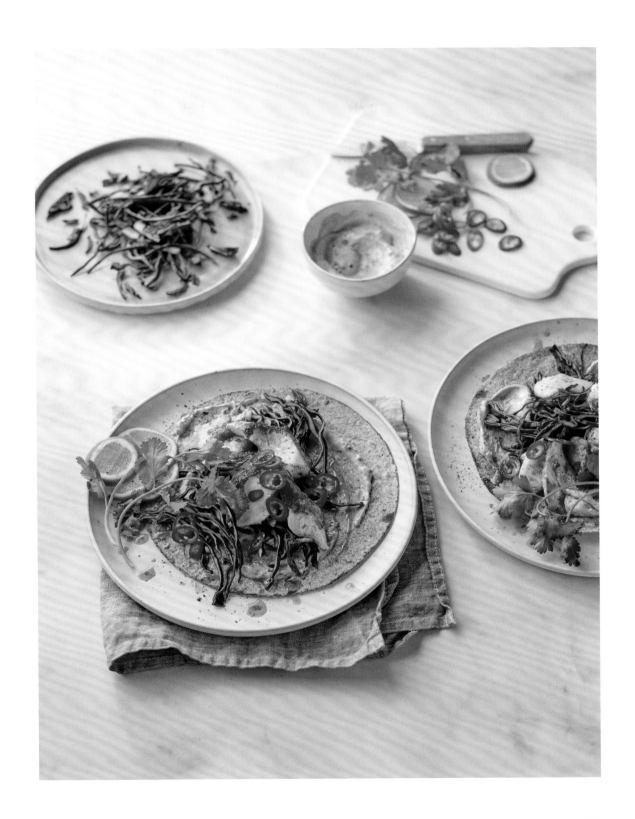

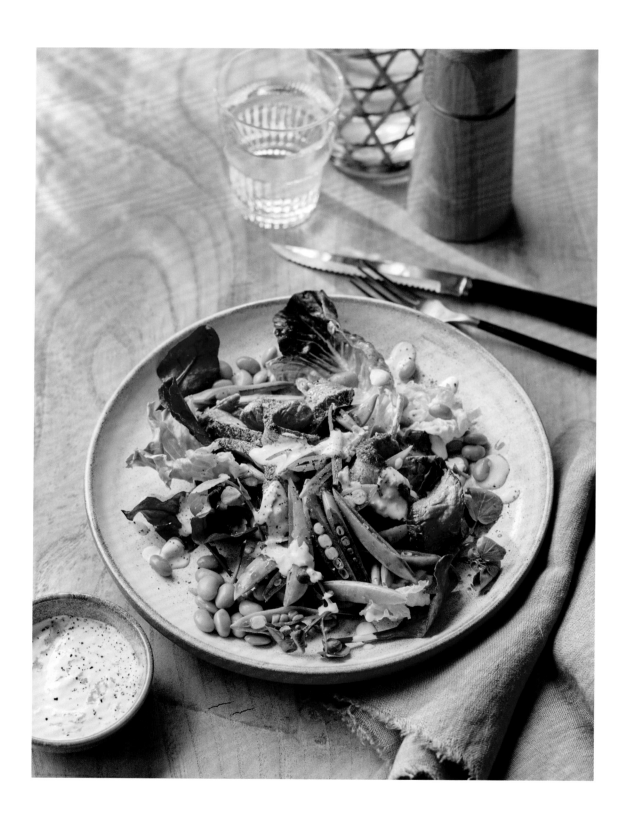

steak & horseradish salad with watercress

serves 2

160g (5½oz) fillet steak
½ tablespoon rapeseed oil
150g (5½oz) edamame (soya)
  beans, shelled
120g (4¼oz) mixed leaves
  (watercress, spinach, rocket,
  baby leaves)
100g (3½oz) sugar snap peas,
  sliced on the diagonal
sea salt and freshly ground
  pepper

for the dressing

1 tablespoon hot horseradish
  sauce
2 tablespoons Greek or live
  natural yogurt
1 teaspoon agave syrup
zest and juice of ½ lemon
sea salt and freshly ground
  pepper

And you thought you couldn't have steak and fast. Good news, everyone – you can. Packed with iron and protein, this cut is low on fat, but high on flavour. The horseradish is a tried and tested combination, of course, while the rocket gives it that little note of bitterness, which is fantastic for stimulating digestion.

Heat a griddle or frying pan over a high heat. Brush the steak with the oil on both sides and season well. Cook the steak for about 2–3 minutes on each side for medium-rare or a little longer if you like it well-done. Set aside on a plate to rest.

Make the dressing by mixing the horseradish, yogurt, agave syrup and lemon zest and juice in a small bowl, adding some seasoning.

Bring a small pan of water to the boil. Cook the shelled edamame for 2 minutes and then drain.

Divide the leaves between two plates, adding the sugar snap peas, edamame and sliced steak. Drizzle over the dressing.

PREP 10 minutes	COOK 10 minutes	CALORIES 314

gluten
free

dairy
free

700 day

green superfood salad with crispy prosciutto

serves 2

juice of ½ lemon
1 tablespoon Dijon mustard
1 garlic clove, grated
2 tablespoons olive oil
200g (7oz) kale or cavolo nero,
  stalks removed and finely
  sliced
150g (5½oz) Brussels sprouts,
  shredded or very finely sliced
3 slices of prosciutto
20g (¾oz) walnuts, roughly
  chopped
sea salt and freshly ground
  pepper

This salad might actually make you cleverer, which is unexpected for just a salad, but that's walnuts for you. Walnuts are a superfood for the brain, as they are full of omega 3 and polyphenols – plant chemicals that reduce inflammation and improve mental clarity. This recipe is also a veritable cruciferous vegetable celebration, with antioxidants that support liver function and immunity like you wouldn't believe.

Add the lemon juice, mustard, garlic and half the olive oil to a little bowl, mixing them together until combined. Add a touch of seasoning to taste.

Heat the rest of the oil in a frying pan over a medium heat and add the kale or cavolo nero and Brussels sprouts. Flash-fry them for a couple of minutes at most as you want them to keep their crunch.

Tip them into a largish bowl and return the pan to the heat. Add the prosciutto slices, trying to lay them out as flat as you can, and then fry for a couple of minutes until crispy.

When the prosciutto slices have crisped up, transfer them to some kitchen paper to remove any excess oil. When they have cooled enough to handle, tear them up into strips.

Add the dressing to the bowl of greens and combine. Divide between two plates and serve with the crispy bits of prosciutto and the walnuts scattered over.

medium
calorie

PREP 15 minutes	COOK 5 minutes	CALORIES 313

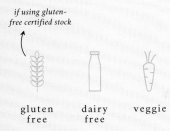

if using gluten-free certified stock

gluten free

dairy free

veggie

spicy kimchi broth with tofu

serves 2

500ml (18fl oz) vegetable stock (shop-bought or home-made)
200g (7oz) firm tofu, cut into small cubes
4 tablespoons kimchi
1 tablespoon sriracha
2 tablespoons tamari
1 head of pak choy, sliced lengthways into strips
2 spring onions, chopped
1 tablespoon sesame oil
2 organic or free-range egg yolks
2 tablespoons toasted sesame seeds
sea salt and freshly ground pepper

If there's one thing the body's microbiome loves, it's a good dose of fermentation. Aside from the tofu (fermented soya) in this recipe, you have kimchi (Korean fermented cabbage), which has taken the fermentation world by storm. If there were a fermented album chart, it would have been number one for years. A low-calorie, vegetable-packed all-round winner.

Heat the stock in a pan over a medium heat, before adding the tofu, kimchi, sriracha, tamari and fish sauce. Let it simmer for 15–20 minutes.

The pak choy goes in next, along with the spring onions and sesame oil. Continue to cook for no more than 1 minute. Give it a taste and season accordingly.

Divide between two bowls and serve with an egg yolk in each one and a sprinkling of sesame seeds.

medium calorie

PREP 5 minutes	COOK 20–25 minutes	CALORIES 334

gluten
free

dairy
free

100 day

lemon & quinoa-crusted sea bass with asparagus

serves 2

250g (9oz) asparagus, lower,
   woodier part of the stems
   snapped off
1 teaspoon chilli flakes
1 teaspoon garlic powder
2 tablespoons olive oil
100g (3½oz) quinoa flakes
1 tablespoon lemon zest
1 organic or free-range egg
2 sea bass fillets (approx.
   180g/6½oz each)
sea salt and freshly ground
   pepper

to serve

1 tablespoon chopped flat-leaf
   parsley
lemon juice

Think fish and chips – but better. And adding quinoa flakes takes the protein content to new heights. Quinoa flakes are slightly different to the grain that most people are familiar with; and should be available in most good health food stores or online. They give the fish a slightly crunchy crust – and what's not to love about that? In place of the chips, we have asparagus instead – little green stalks of vitamins A, C and K, plus folate, fibre and prebiotics, which feed the bacteria in the intestine. Joyful.

Preheat the oven to 220°C (425°F), Gas Mark 7.

Line a baking tray with baking paper and add the asparagus, mixing it with the chilli flakes, garlic powder and half the olive oil. Roast in the oven for 10–12 minutes.

While the asparagus is in the oven, combine the quinoa flakes with the lemon zest in a wide bowl or on a plate. Beat the egg in a separate (preferably shallow and wide) bowl. Dip each fish fillet into the egg mixture before dipping it into the quinoa flake mixture, so that it's coated on both sides. Season well.

Heat the remaining oil in a frying pan over a medium heat and fry the fish on each side for about 2–3 minutes, depending on its thickness. You want it to look crispy and golden.

Serve with the roasted asparagus, a sprinkling of parsley and a spritz of lemon juice.

medium
calorie

PREP 10 minutes	COOK 20 minutes	CALORIES 507

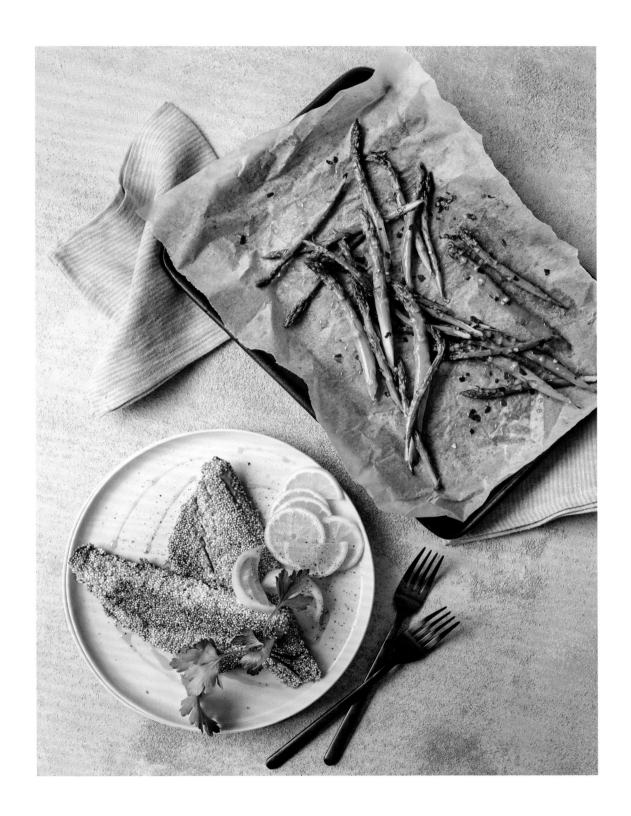

gluten
free

dairy
free

vegan

100 day

power pot: butterbean, chickpea & cherry tomato

serves 1

¼ can (100g/3½oz) can of butter beans, drained and rinsed
¼ can (100g/3½oz) can of chickpeas, drained and rinsed
6 cherry tomatoes, halved
4 radishes, quartered
20g (¾oz) spinach, shredded
¼ red onion, finely chopped
½ tablespoon olive oil
2 teaspoons apple cider vinegar
10g (¼oz) parsley, chopped
splash of water to thin the dressing, if necessary
sea salt and freshly ground pepper

I love a protein-packed power pot with beans and grains, but this recipe and the one on page 148 are very flexible – just have a dig around, see what vegetables you have hanging around and add them to the mix. Easy.

Add all the ingredients to a bowl and mix thoroughly, seasoning to taste. Transfer to a covered container or lidded jar and chill in the refrigerator overnight before serving.

medium
calorie

PREP 5 minutes	CHILL overnight	CALORIES 311

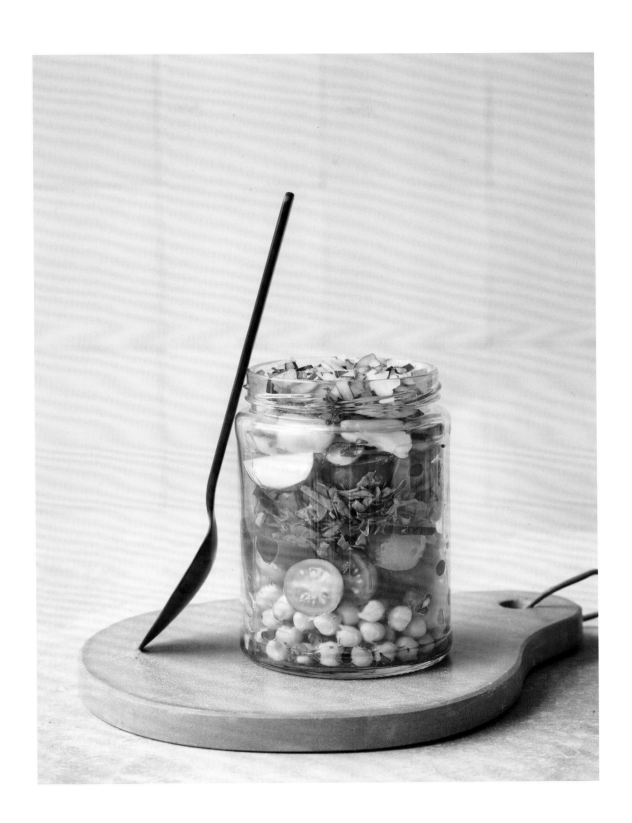

gluten
free

dairy
free

vegan

power pot: avocado & edamame superfood

serves 1

80g (3oz) frozen shelled
   edamame (soya) beans
flesh of ½ ripe avocado, chopped
1 tablespoon mixed sprouted
   grains (chickpea, lentil, alfalfa)
2 tablespoons cooked quinoa
   (from a precooked packet)
1 teaspoon apple cider vinegar
½ tablespoon tamari
½ tablespoon yuzu ponzu
   seasoning
juice of ½ lime
sea salt and freshly ground
   pepper

Sprouted grains, edamame beans, avocado and quinoa
– a crunchy and delicious combination of protein, healthy
fats and concentrated nutrients all brought to life with
a vibrant citrussy dressing. A light, but satisfying lunch
to stabilise blood sugar levels and keep energy flowing
through the day.

Add all the ingredients to a bowl and mix thoroughly,
seasoning to taste. Transfer to a covered container or lidded
jar and chill in the refrigerator overnight before serving.

medium
calorie

| PREP 5 minutes | COOK overnight | CALORIES 312 |

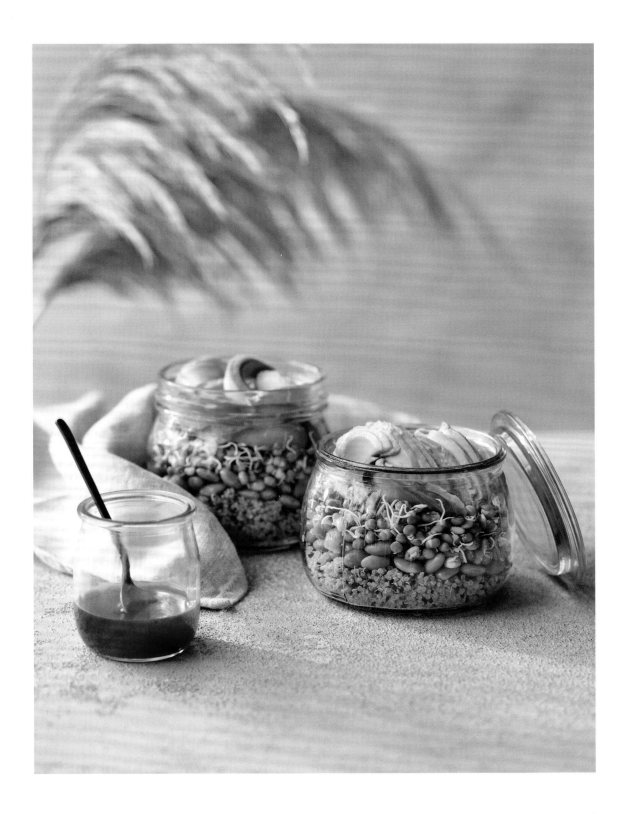

gluten
free

dairy
free

veggie

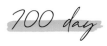

healthy poké bowl

serves 2

2 organic or free-range eggs, at
   room temperature
iced water
200g (7oz) long-stem broccoli,
   ends trimmed and chopped
1 tablespoon rapeseed oil
1 tablespoons cold-pressed oil
   (flaxseed, hemp seed, pumpkin
   seed, extra virgin olive)
1 small shallot, finely chopped
1 tablespoon apple cider vinegar
½ tablespoon Dijon mustard
½ small cabbage, shredded
   (savoy, hispi, cavolo nero)
100g (3½oz) baby spinach
6 radishes, thinly sliced
flesh of ½ ripe avocado, sliced
1 tablespoon pumpkin seeds
sea salt and freshly ground
   pepper

Poké bowls are all the rage right now and for good reason.
They are typically made with raw fish, rice and lots of other
delectable ingredients, but this version takes the calories
right down without compromising on deliciousness. Very
simple to make, it has great protein and vitamin B content
thanks to the eggs, plus lovely healthy fats from the
avocado. The apple cider vinegar in the dressing is high in
polyphenols, is a fantastic cleanser for the body and helps
to balance blood sugar levels. Clever!

Preheat the oven to 220°C (425°F), Gas Mark 7 and line a
baking tray with foil.

Bring a pan of water to the boil. Add the eggs and cook
for 6 minutes so that the whites have set but the yolks are
still runny.

Carefully remove the eggs and briefly hold them under cold
running water before adding them to a bowl of iced water.
Once they're cool enough to handle, peel them and cut
them in half. Then set aside.

Add the broccoli with the rapeseed oil to the foil-lined tray,
season and then mix together to coat. Roast in the oven for
10 minutes. While that's happening, prepare the dressing by
combining the cold-pressed with the shallot, vinegar and
mustard, and then season to taste.

Add the cabbage and spinach to a largish bowl and combine
with the dressing, rubbing it into the cabbage leaves to
soften them a little. Then add the broccoli, radishes, avocado,
pumpkin seeds and eggs, and serve.

medium
calorie

PREP 15 minutes	COOK 20 minutes	CALORIES 387

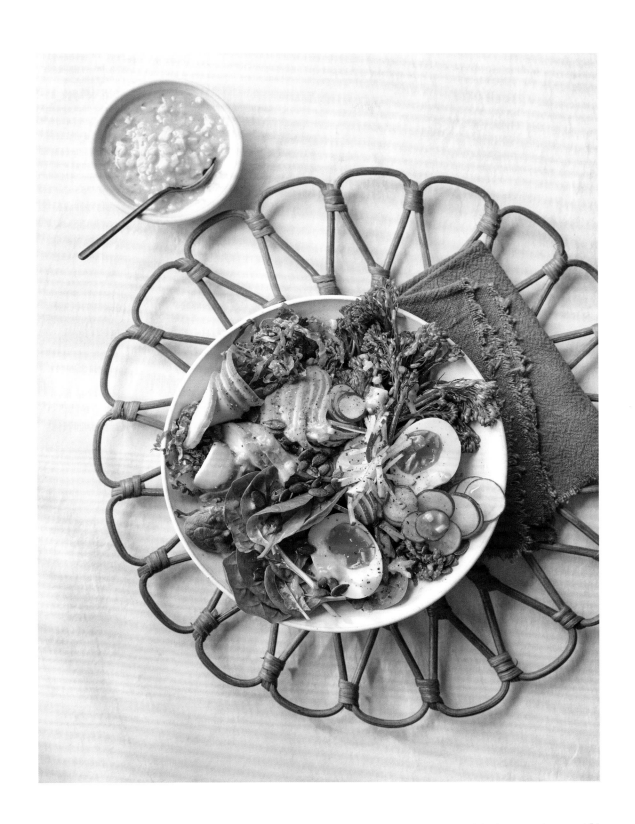

700 day

pink & green salad of dreams

serves 2

for the salad

150g (5½oz) organic or free-range chicken breast or roasted, shop-bought chicken
juice of ½ lemon
¼ teaspoon chilli flakes
2 tablespoons pumpkin seeds
80g (3oz) Little Gem lettuce leaves
1 Chioggia beetroot, scrubbed and thinly sliced
2 tablespoons sprouted seeds (alfalfa, broccoli, radish, kale)
sea salt and freshly ground pepper

for the dressing

3 tablespoons Greek or live natural yogurt
1 garlic clove, grated
1 tablespoon sriracha
juice of ½ lemon

to serve

2 tablespoons pomegranate seeds
1 tablespoon finely chopped flat-leaf parsley
sea salt and ground pepper

super-low cal

The only problem with this salad is that it's so good-looking, you might just want to Instagram it instead of eating it. The beetroot looks like candy cane but is a great deal healthier, I can assure you, and the pomegranate seeds add tiny bursts of bright sweetness. Pink and green are the dream colour combination and this salad is like art – art you can eat that also has anti-inflammatory properties to keep you feeling energised and sprightly.

Place the raw chicken breasts (if using) on a piece of foil big enough to fold into a biggish parcel. Squeeze over the lemon juice, sprinkle over the chilli flakes and season well. Fold up the sides and seal together to form a loose parcel around the chicken. Place on a baking tray and bake for around 30–35 minutes. Once cooked, set aside to cool before tearing into strips or chunks. If using shop-bought roast chicken, squeeze over the lemon juice, sprinkle over the chilli flakes, season well and tear into strips.

Heat a frying pan over a medium heat and add the pumpkin seeds (you don't need any oil). Fry them, constantly stirring, until they start popping, which will happen pretty quickly. Then set aside to cool.

Add the lettuce and beetroot to a salad bowl, along with the sprouted seeds, chicken and pumpkin seeds.

To make the dressing, place all the ingredients in a small bowl and then mix well. Pour it over the salad and toss. Serve with the pomegranate seeds and parsley and season.

PREP 10 minutes	COOK 35–40 minutes	CALORIES 240

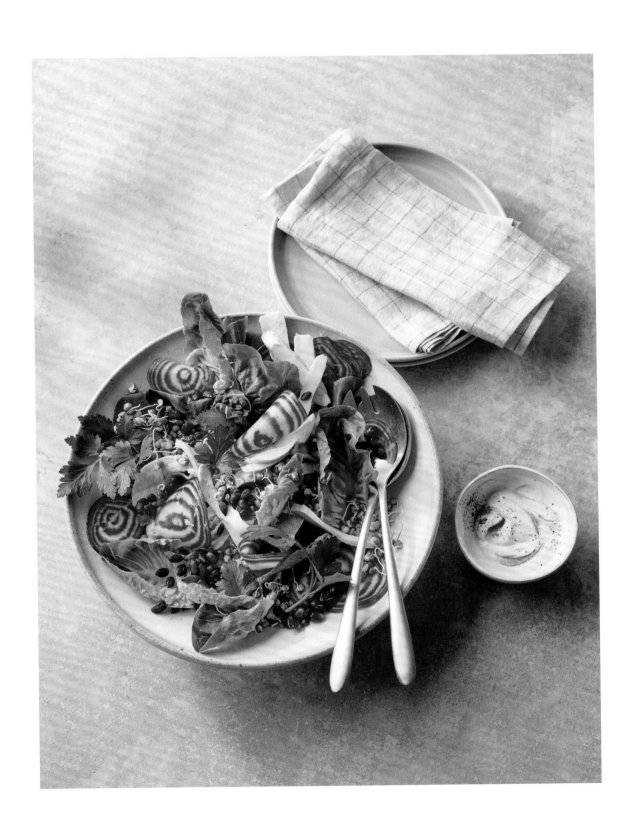

if using gluten-free certified miso

gluten free   dairy free   vegan

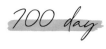
100 day

grilled miso aubergines

serves 2

for the aubergines
2 aubergines, halved lengthways
½ tablespoon olive oil
sea salt and freshly ground
  pepper

for the paste
2 tablespoons white miso paste
2 tablespoons mirin
1 tablespoon tamari
1 teaspoon agave syrup
1 teaspoon sesame oil

to serve
1 teaspoon black sesame seeds
½ red chilli, deseeded and thinly
  sliced
a few fresh coriander sprigs

With a purple skin rich in anthocyanins, aubergines are a good source of antioxidants. They're high in fibre, which makes them lovely and filling, but low in calories. The delicious, sweet East-Asian ingredients pack them full of flavour – try serving with crunchy lettuce leaves spritzed with lime juice.

Preheat the oven to 220°C (425°F), Gas Mark 7, and line a baking tray with foil.

Sprinkle the four aubergine halves with salt. Leave them for 15 minutes to drain off some of the excess water. Then wash off the salt and pat them dry.

Using a sharp knife, score the flesh of the aubergines in a criss-cross pattern, going as deep as you can but being careful not to pierce the skin. Brush them with the olive oil and place them on the foil-lined tray. Bake for about 30 minutes or until the flesh is soft.

While the aubergines are in the oven, make up the paste. Place the miso, mirin, tamari, agave syrup and sesame oil into a mixing bowl and mix well. Set aside.

Remove the aubergines from the oven (leave the oven on as they'll be going back in). Allow them to cool for a few minutes and then carefully scoop the flesh out using a spoon. Add it to the bowl with the paste and mix everything together, then spoon the mixture back into the aubergine skins.

Return the aubergines to the oven for a further 5 minutes until they are lovely and hot. Serve with a sprinkling of sesame seeds, red chilli and a few coriander leaves.

super-low cal

PREP 25 minutes	COOK 35 minutes	CALORIES 196

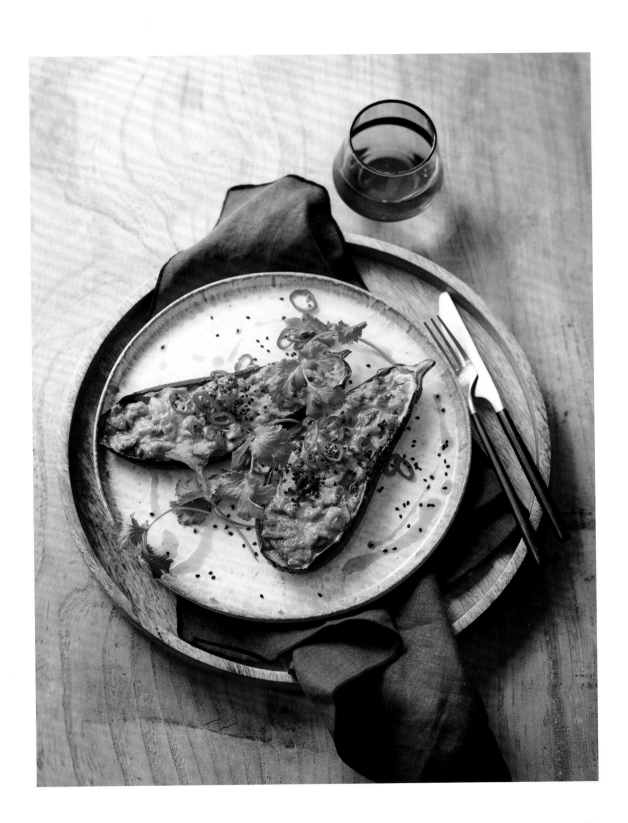

gluten
free

100 day

chicory salad with goats' cheese & pancetta croutons

serves 4

for the salad

40g (1½oz) diced pancetta
1 small or ½ large radicchio,
  leaves separated and washed
1 white chicory head, leaves
  separated and washed
1 bag rocket (approx. 60g/2¼oz)
70g (2½oz) your favourite goats'
  cheese, cubed, crumbled, grated
  or sliced
40g (1½oz) walnut halves
sea salt and freshly ground
  pepper

for the dressing

2 tablespoons apple cider
  vinegar
4 tablespoons cold-pressed oil
  (flaxseed, hemp seed, pumpkin
  seed, extra virgin olive)
½ teaspoon Dijon mustard
½ shallot, finely chopped
squeeze of agave syrup, to taste

The bitterness of chicory and radicchio is a fantastic stimulant for the digestive system, which not only helps break down the creamy goats' cheese and salty pancetta, but also balances perfectly as a flavour combination. Crunchy walnuts are famously good for the brain, containing phytochemicals and healthy fats – so yes, this salad may not only leave you feeling surprisingly intelligent, it's very likely to put you in a really good mood.

Preheat the oven to 200°C (400°F), Gas Mark 6.

Line a baking tray with foil and scatter the pancetta over, breaking up any clumps. Roast in the oven for about 20 minutes or until golden and crispy. Then set aside to cool a little.

Place the radicchio, chicory and rocket in a large bowl, followed by the cheese, most of the walnuts and the cooled pancetta. Mix thoroughly.

Whisk all the dressing ingredients together in a bowl and then drizzle over the salad. Add the remaining walnuts as a garnish.

super-low
cal

| PREP 10 minutes | COOK 20 minutes | CALORIES 295 |

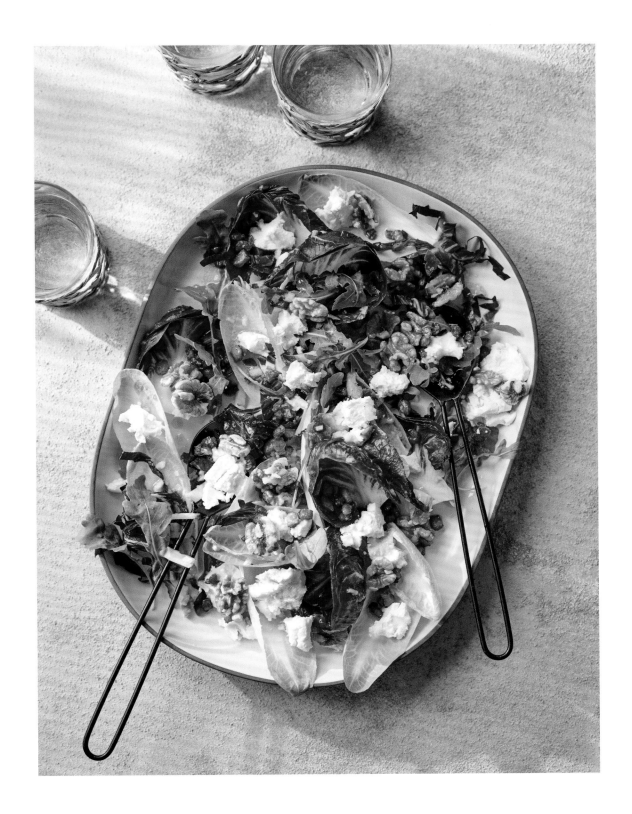

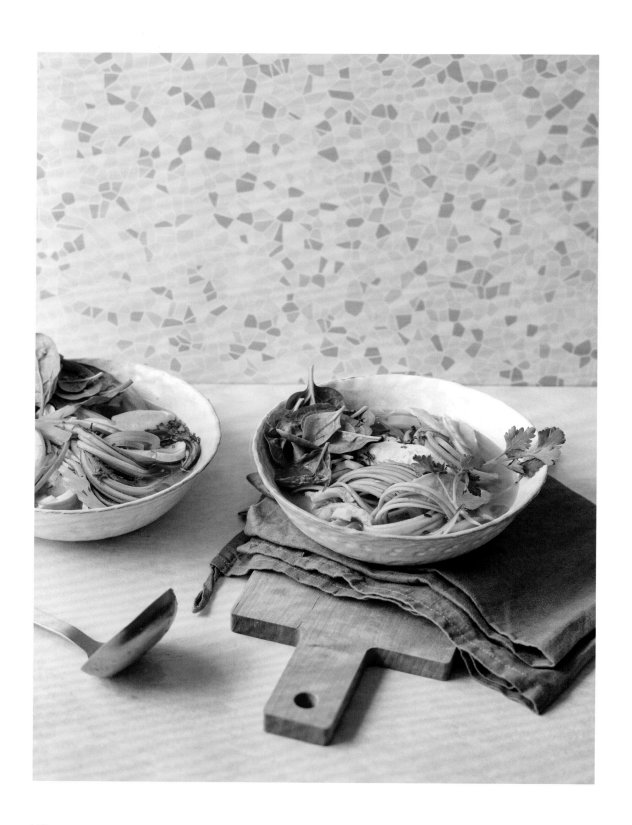

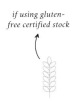
700 day

warming chicken soup with ginger & courgette

serves 2

1 large organic or free-range
  chicken breast (approx.
  180g/6½oz) or chicken left
  over from a roast
1 tablespoon olive oil
2cm (¾-inch) piece of fresh
  ginger, peeled and grated
2 garlic cloves, grated
1 teaspoon ground turmeric
500ml (18fl oz) chicken stock
  (shop-bought or home-made)
2 celery sticks, thinly sliced
1 carrot, spiralised or cut into
  thin strips
handful of spinach (approx.
  30g/1oz)
½ teaspoon cayenne pepper
juice of ½ lime
1 large courgette, spiralised or
  cut into thin strips
sea salt and freshly ground
  pepper

to serve
chopped parsley
1 teaspoon chilli oil, for
  drizzling (optional)

If you've ever found yourself looking at the remnants of a roast chicken and thinking, 'What am I supposed to do with you now?', here's your answer. Chicken broth is one of those dishes that it's impossible not to be comforted by – and adding ginger and cayenne pepper gives it a bit of heat, which is important during fasting. It's not all about salads, you know.

If using raw chicken breast, heat a pan of water until simmering. Add the chicken breast and poach for 10–12 minutes or until cooked through. Remove from the heat and set aside.

In the meantime, heat the oil in a pan over a medium heat and add the ginger, garlic and turmeric. Then add the stock and simmer for 15–20 minutes.

Shred the now cooled chicken – or any leftover chicken, if you're using that – and add to the broth. Next, add the celery and carrot and heat them through for just a couple of minutes, if you want to keep them crunchy. Stir in the spinach until it has wilted. Add the cayenne pepper, lime juice and seasoning.

Divide the courgette between two bowls and ladle over the broth, along with a sprinkling of parsley and a swirl of chilli oil (if using).

super-low
cal

PREP 20 minutes	COOK 20–35 minutes	CALORIES 263 (without chilli oil) 303 (with chilli oil)

if using gluten-free certified stock

gluten
free

dairy
free

700 day

leafy detox pho with prawns

serves 2

1 tablespoon coconut oil
1 teaspoon coriander seeds,
  crushed
2 cardamom seeds, crushed
1 teaspoon Chinese five spice
2cm (¾-inch) piece of fresh ginger,
  thinly sliced (unpeeled)
2 garlic cloves, grated
475ml (17fl oz) bone stock
  (shop-bought or home-made)
120g (4¼oz) mushrooms, sliced
  (shiitake, oyster, wild, porcini)
1 star anise
1 cinnamon stick
1 tablespoon fish sauce
1 tablespoon tamari
200g (7oz) zero-calorie konjac
  noodles
2 handfuls of leafy greens of your
  choice (chard, spinach, kale)
200g (7oz) raw peeled prawns
juice of 1 lime
sea salt and freshly ground pepper

to serve

1 red chilli, deseeded and thinly
  sliced
75g (2½oz) bean sprouts
1 spring onion, thinly sliced
1 small carrot, grated
Thai basil, roughly torn
fresh coriander, chopped

super-low
cal

This warming detox pho is fragrant with Chinese spices and has the added bonus of succulent prawns and plenty of nutrient-rich vegetables. The sort of dish that instantly cheers your spirits, it's delicious with all kinds of noodles – but for the purposes of fasting, it's important to stick to the zero-calorie variety, which are available online or in health food shops. On a mindful day, however, all bets are off.

Heat the coconut oil in a pan over a medium heat and add the coriander seeds, cardamom seeds and Chinese five spice. Keep them moving for a minute or so until they become lovely and fragrant. Add the ginger and garlic and stir for another minute before adding the stock, mushrooms, star anise, cinnamon stick, fish sauce and tamari. Bring it to the boil before reducing to a simmer and letting it cook, uncovered, for about 15–20 minutes.

Carefully remove the star anise and cinnamon and taste to see if you want to add any more fish sauce, tamari or some seasoning. Cover with a lid and keep it over a low heat.

Prepare the noodles according to the packet instructions and divide between two bowls.

Bring the broth back up to a simmer, add the leafy greens and let them wilt, followed by the prawns and lime juice. Cook the prawns until they turn pink (should be about 2 minutes or so) and then take the broth off the heat. Ladle into the two bowls of noodles and add whichever serving suggestions look the most appetising to you in the moment.

PREP 20 minutes	COOK 30–35 minutes	CALORIES 240

gluten
free

veggie

halloumi, pepper & beetroot salad

serves 2

for the dressing

1 tablespoon Dijon mustard
1 teaspoon agave syrup
½ tablespoon apple cider vinegar
1 tablespoon rapeseed or olive
   oil

for the salad

100g (3½oz) watercress
1 yellow pepper, cored, deseeded
   and sliced lengthways
35g (1¼oz) grated or sliced
   pickled beetroot
110g (4oz) halloumi, sliced
1 tablespoon pine nuts, to serve

Halloumi – that delicious, straight-off-the-grill flavour – always makes me think of being on holiday in Greece and taking a break from the beach for lunch. Apart from transporting you under a Grecian sun, halloumi is a good source of protein. Along with the antioxidant benefits of beetroot, this light salad has the added joy of being extremely quick to make.

Mix up the mustard, agave syrup, apple cider vinegar and rapeseed oil together in a small bowl to make the dressing. Then set aside.

Place the watercress, pepper and beetroot on a large plate or in a bowl and mix together. Then add the dressing and toss to mix.

Heat a griddle or frying pan over a medium heat and add the halloumi slices. Cook for about 3 minutes or until golden on each side. Add them to the rest of the salad and finish with a sprinkling of pine nuts.

super-low
cal

PREP 10 minutes	COOK 10 minutes	CALORIES 331

gluten
free

dairy
free

vegan

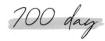
100 day

vegetable crisps

serves 2

1 sweet potato
1 large carrot
2 beetroots
2 tablespoons olive oil
1 teaspoon ground fennel seeds
½ teaspoon cayenne pepper
sea salt and freshly ground
 pepper

A sweeter version of their greasy potato cousin, vegetable crisps are a much healthier alternative to the kind of crisps you might throw into your basket at the supermarket. Packed with longevity-loving phytonutrients, they are baked rather than fried, trans-fats-free (try saying that after three martinis) – and, incidentally, really good with martinis.

Preheat the oven to 200°C (400°F), Gas Mark 6 and line a large baking tray with foil.

Peel or scrub the vegetables and then slice as thinly as possible using a sharp knife or peeler. Pat them dry before adding the olive oil, ground fennel seeds, cayenne pepper and seasoning.

Add the vegetables in groups to the baking tray and spread them out as much as you can. Separating them means that if some start to cook faster than the others, it will be easier to remove them earlier. Roast for 10–15 minutes before turning and then roasting for a further 5 minutes.

Remove from the oven and let them cool on a wire rack so they can crisp up. Eat on their own or with your favourite dip.

super-low
cal

PREP 10 minutes	COOK 15–20 minutes	CALORIES 238

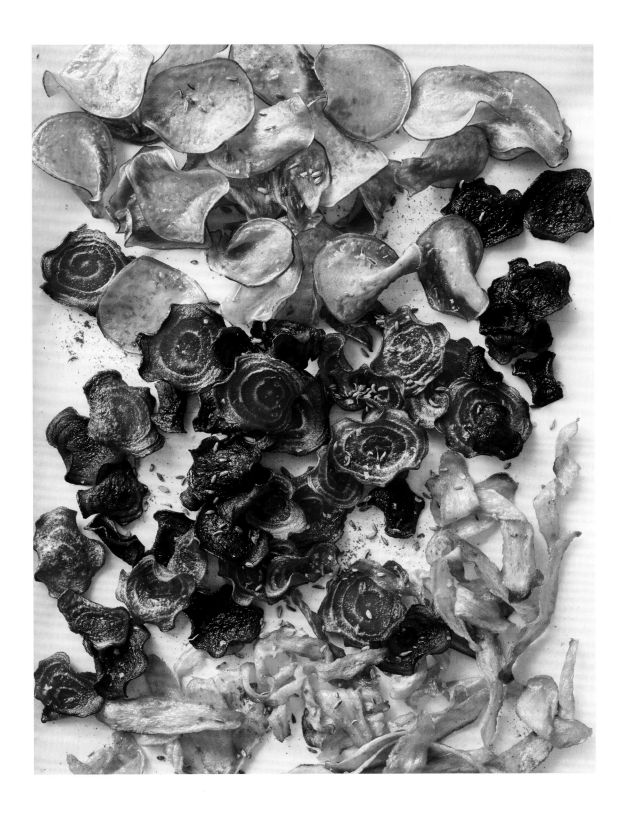

gluten
free

dairy
free

vegan

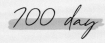

crunchy roasted chickpeas

serves 2

400g (14oz) can of chickpeas,
    drained and rinsed (240g/8½oz
    drained weight)
½ tablespoon olive oil
1 tablespoon apple cider vinegar
sea salt and freshly ground
    pepper

Apart from being an amazing, healthy snack, roasted chickpeas are also really delicious in salads as an alternative to croutons. Again, the flavour options are endless, from lime and cracked pepper to dark chocolate, so don't hold back. Chickpeas are very high in soluble fibre, which will keep your digestion happy and also help reduce any feelings of hunger. They're also an excellent alternative source of protein for vegetarians and vegans. You'll never bother with popcorn again.

Preheat the oven to 200°C (400°F), Gas Mark 6.

Pat the chickpeas dry with a tea towel – this will help them crisp up properly.

Add the oil, season generously and mix well to ensure the chickpeas are coated before tipping them onto a baking tray. Roast for 20 minutes and then give the tray a shake and cook for a further 10 minutes.

Remove from the oven, add the vinegar and toss, then return to the oven for 1 minute; they should emerge golden and crunchy. Leave to cool and store in an airtight container.

super-low
cal

| PREP 5 minutes | COOK 30 minutes | CALORIES 161 |

gluten
free

dairy
free

vegan

crispy kale chips

serves 2

250g (9oz) kale leaves, stems
  removed and roughly chopped
1 tablespoon olive oil
½ teaspoon smoked paprika
1½ teaspoons garlic powder
¾ teaspoon chilli flakes
½ tablespoon sesame seeds
sea salt and freshly ground
  pepper

Welcome to my all-time favourite snack. Kale chips are outrageously good, but I highly recommend making them with cavolo nero, which I almost prefer. They work with lots of different seasoning options – tahini, Parmesan or nutritional yeast (the vegetarian/vegan option instead of Parmesan cheese), Chinese five spice or crushed cashew nuts and lemon juice, to name a few. The options are endless, so have a little nose around the internet and get creative. A little aside – kale chips are very easy to burn or undercook, as everyone's oven is different, so keep an eye on yours for the first couple of batches.

Preheat the oven to 150°C (300°F), Gas Mark 2, and line a baking tray with nonstick baking paper.

Wash the kale leaves thoroughly, dry them and then tip them into a large bowl. Add the oil and massage it into the leaves so that they're coated, albeit lightly (add a little more oil if you really think it needs it, but the aim is to keep the oil to a minimum as this will help the kale crisp up).

Add the smoked paprika, garlic powder, chilli flakes, sesame seeds and seasoning, mixing everything together thoroughly so the spices are evenly distributed. Spread the kale out in a shallow layer on the baking tray. (You may need to do more than one batch, depending on the size of your baking tray).

Roast the kale for 10 minutes, then give it a stir and roast for a further 15 minutes. Kale chips can burn in a flash, so just to remind you, it's a good idea to keep an eye on them. Remove from the oven and leave to cool for 3 minutes to encourage further crisping before tucking in.

super-low
cal

PREP 15 minutes	COOK 25 minutes	CALORIES 128

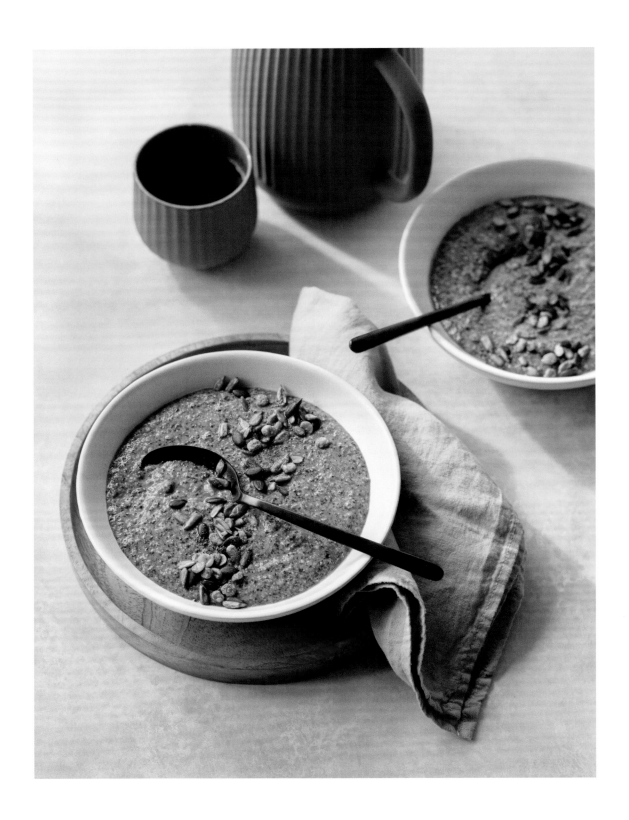

if using gluten-free certified stock

gluten free   dairy free   vegan

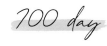

700 day

edamame & broccoli soup

serves 2

½ tablespoon coconut oil
2 spring onions, finely chopped
2 garlic cloves, grated
150g (5½oz) frozen shelled
   edamame (soya) beans
½ head of broccoli (approx.
   200g/7oz), cut into florets and
   stalk trimmed and chopped
150g (5½oz) dark leafy cabbage,
   shredded
500ml (18fl oz) vegetable stock
   (shop-bought or home-made)
juice of ½ lime
sea salt and freshly ground
   pepper
1 tablespoon mixed seeds, to
   serve

Vitamin K, folate, fibre and protein. This is the CV that comes with edamame. And if I fan-girled over broccoli any more than I already do, I would be arrested for public disturbance. The king of the cruciferous vegetable family, its active compounds including flavonoids are known to reduce inflammation. The high antioxidant levels and fibre content of this soup will really help control blood sugar levels, so your body can get on with the important job of getting younger.

Heat the oil in a pan over a medium heat. Add the spring onions and fry for a couple of minutes before adding the garlic for another minute. Next up are the edamame, broccoli, cabbage and stock – bring to the boil and then reduce the heat. Leave to simmer for about 20 minutes.

Remove from the heat and add the lime juice before using a stick blender or pouring into a blender and blitzing until smooth (you may need to do this in batches, depending on the size of your blender). Season and serve with a sprinkling of crunchy seeds.

super-low cal vegan soup

PREP 10 minutes	COOK 25 minutes	CALORIES 253

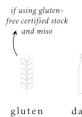

if using gluten-free certified stock and miso

gluten
free

dairy
free

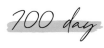

vegan

700 day

vibrant vegetable soup with quinoa

serves 2

½ tablespoon coconut oil
1 shallot, chopped
1 celery stick, sliced
1 parsnip, chopped
1 carrot, chopped
30g (1oz) dry quinoa
800ml (27fl oz) vegetable stock
  (shop-bought or home-made)
1 tablespoon white miso paste
½ head (260g/9oz) cauliflower,
  chopped
2 garlic cloves, grated
2cm (¾-inch) piece of fresh
  ginger, peeled and grated
1 red chilli, deseeded and finely
  sliced
pinch of paprika
large handful of kale (approx.
  30g/1oz), stalks removed and
  roughly chopped
large handful of spinach (approx.
  30g/1oz)
sea salt and freshly ground
  pepper

With plenty of nutrient-rich vegetables, this soup is very good for digestion and will leave you feeling fuller than you might think. The fermented properties in the miso and high fibre content will feed good bacteria in the intestinal tract, while the low calorie count will help support the body in its state of autophagy.

Heat the oil in a pan (preferably with a lid) over a medium heat. Next, add the shallot, celery, parsnip and carrot and gently fry for about 8 minutes, stirring every now and then so that the vegetables colour a little but don't catch.

Add the quinoa, stock, miso, cauliflower, garlic, ginger and chilli and bring to the boil. Reduce the heat to a simmer, cover and cook for about 10–12 minutes.

Finally, add the paprika, kale and spinach and let them wilt – this shouldn't take more than a couple of minutes. Season well and serve.

super-low
cal vegan
soups

PREP 15 minutes	COOK 25 minutes	CALORIES 260

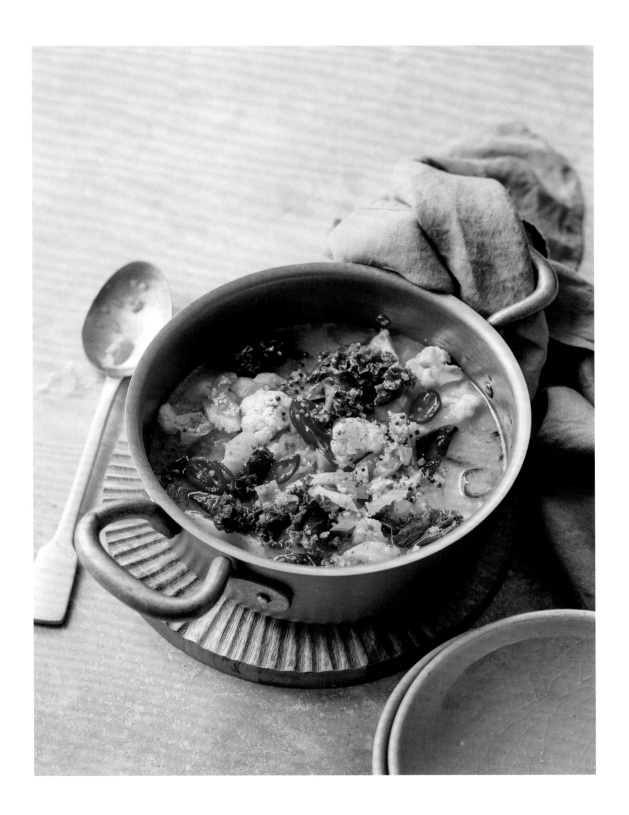

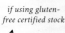

if using gluten-free certified stock

gluten free   dairy free   vegan

100 day

cauliflower, almond & cayenne pepper soup

serves 2

½ tablespoon rapeseed oil
1 onion, finely chopped
2 garlic cloves, grated
½ teaspoon ground nutmeg
zest and juice of ½ lemon
130g (4½oz) cauliflower, cored, cut into small florets, stem chopped, divided
30g (1oz) ground almonds
800ml (27fl oz) vegetable stock (shop-bought or home-made)
sea salt and freshly ground pepper

to serve

¼ teaspoon cayenne pepper or ½ teaspoon chilli oil
20g (¾oz) flaked almonds (roasted or raw)
chopped chives

Cauliflower is the toast of the cruciferous world. If people aren't turning it into rice, they're roasting it as steaks and everything else in between. Texturally, it makes this a dreamy, creamy soup, to which I've added almonds. They not only make it a little more filling, but they also bring magnesium, protein, good fats and vitamin E to the party, the latter two being particularly beneficial for the brain and heart.

Heat the oil in a large pan over a medium heat. Gently cook the onion for about 7 minutes or until softened.

Add the garlic, nutmeg and lemon zest and juice and cook for a further 1 minute. Then add the cauliflower, ground almonds and stock. Season well. Bring to the boil and then reduce to a simmer. Cook for about 20 minutes or until the cauliflower is nice and tender.

Remove from the heat to cool a little. Then add to a blender or use a stick blender and blitz until creamy and smooth (you may need to do this in batches, depending on the size of your blender).

Serve with cayenne pepper or a swirl of chilli oil, crunchy flaked almonds and a sprinkling of chives.

super-low cal vegan soup

PREP 10 minutes	COOK 30 minutes	CALORIES 237

if using gluten-free certified stock

gluten free   dairy free   vegan

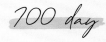
700 day

moroccan-spiced chickpea soup

serves 2

½ tablespoon rapeseed oil
½ onion, chopped
1 carrot, finely chopped
100g (3½oz) sweet potato, chopped into small cubes
2 garlic cloves, grated
1 teaspoon cayenne pepper
1 teaspoon ground cumin
1 teaspoon ground cinnamon
400ml (14fl oz) vegetable stock (shop-bought or home-made)
200g (7oz) canned chopped tomatoes
½ can (200g/7oz) of chickpeas, drained and rinsed
large handful of spinach (approx. 30g/1oz)
juice of ½ lime
sea salt and freshly ground pepper

To serve
fresh coriander, chopped
red chilli flakes

Fragrant with the spices of Morocco, this soup is an excellent source of vegan protein, thanks to the chickpeas – a staple ingredient of classic Middle Eastern dishes. The tomatoes are rich in the antioxidant lycopene and bring a depth of flavour, while the sweet potato delivers a lovely earthy kick.

Heat the oil in a pan over a medium heat. Add the onion, carrot and sweet potato and fry for about 10 minutes, stirring often.

Add the garlic, cayenne pepper, cumin and cinnamon and fry for another minute until the spices are fragrant. Next, add the stock, tomatoes and chickpeas and simmer for about 8 minutes.

Stir in the spinach so it can wilt for a minute. Add the lime juice and season before serving.

super-low cal vegan soup

PREP 10 minutes	COOK 20 minutes	CALORIES 270

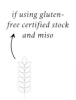

*if using gluten-
free certified stock
and miso*

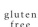

gluten
free

dairy
free

vegan

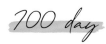

100 day

asian mushroom & miso ramen

serves 2

650ml (22fl oz) vegetable stock
  (shop-bought or home-made)
1 garlic clove, grated
3cm (1¼-inch) piece of fresh
  ginger, peeled and grated
1 red chilli, deseeded and sliced
3 lime leaves
2 tablespoons miso paste, red or
  white according to preference
200g (7oz) zero-calorie konjac
  noodles
½ tablespoon coconut oil
3 spring onions, sliced
125g (4½oz) shiitake mushrooms,
  sliced
2 pak choy, leaves sliced in half
  lengthways
small handful of Thai basil
  leaves (approx. 20g/¾oz), torn
2 tablespoon tamari
1 teaspoon sesame oil
30g (1oz) bean sprouts
juice of 1 lime

to serve

couple of sprigs of fresh
  coriander, chopped
½ red chilli, deseeded and sliced

I am a big fan of soup when it comes to fasting, as you can pack them with low-calorie vegetables, plus they are always comforting and warming. I love shiitake mushrooms, which boost immunity and are high in vitamins B and D, but feel free to substitute them with other mushrooms, if you prefer. They're a family of tiny powerhouses with all kinds of health benefits.

Heat the stock in a pan over a medium heat. Add the garlic, ginger, chilli and lime leaves and stir in the miso. Leave to gently simmer for 10 minutes.

Meanwhile, prepare the noodles according to the packet instructions.

Heat the coconut oil in another pan over a medium-high heat and add the spring onions, mushrooms and pak choy, stirring for about 3 minutes. Then add the Thai basil, fish sauce, soy sauce, sesame oil and bean sprouts and cook for another minute. You want the vegetables to be hot, but still have a crunch to them. Take off the heat, remove the lime leaves and add the lime juice.

Divide the noodles between two warmed bowls and ladle over the vegetable broth. Serve with a few coriander leaves and some slices of red chilli.

super-low
cal vegan
soup

PREP 15 minutes	COOK 20 minutes	CALORIES 152

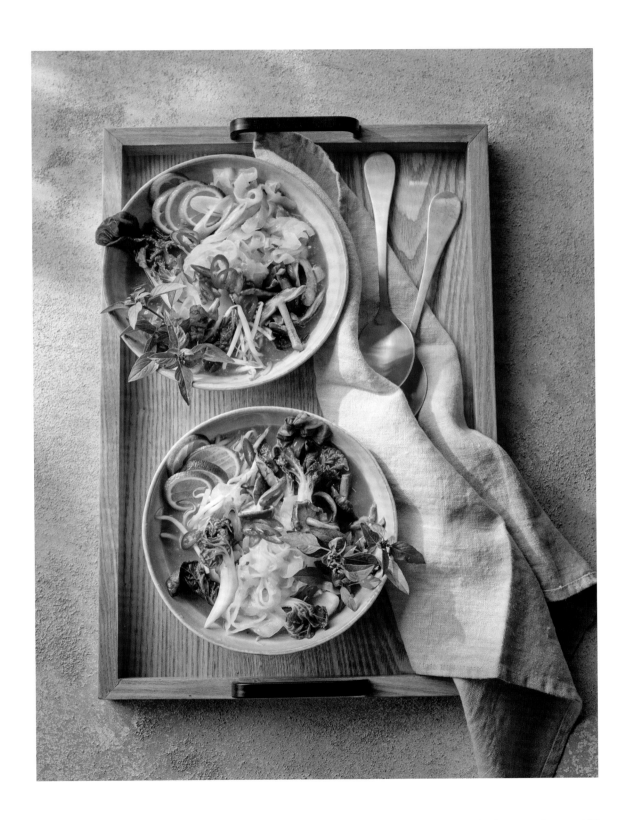

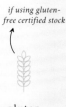

if using gluten-free certified stock

gluten
free

dairy
free

vegan

100 day

thai turmeric soup
with butternut squash

serves 2

This immune-supporting soup blends the flavours of
Thailand with the comforting sweetness of butternut
squash. Spicy ginger and fiery red chilli are balanced with
creamy coconut milk, which is a healthier alternative to
dairy. The best options to go for are organic light coconut
milk or the kind you buy in cartons which is typically
blended with rice milk.

500g (1lb 2oz) deseeded
butternut squash flesh, roughly
chopped
1 tablespoon olive oil
1 garlic clove, grated
2cm (¾-inch) piece of fresh
ginger, peeled and grated
1 red chilli, deseeded and thinly
sliced (put some aside to serve)
1 teaspoon ground turmeric
1 tablespoon Thai red curry
paste
120ml (4fl oz) coconut milk
350ml (12fl oz) vegetable stock
(shop-bought or home-made)
½ tablespoon tamari
½ lemongrass stalk
3 lime leaves
juice of 1 lime
couple of sprigs of fresh
coriander, chopped
sea salt and freshly ground
pepper

Preheat the oven to 200°C (400°F), Gas Mark 6.

Scatter the butternut squash in a roasting tin or on a baking
tray, toss it in half the oil and season well. Roast in the oven
for about 30 minutes until tender.

Heat the rest of the oil in a pan over a medium heat and then
add the garlic, ginger, chilli and turmeric. Gently fry them for
a couple of minutes until fragrant. The Thai red curry paste
goes in next, along with the roasted butternut squash, the
coconut milk, stock, fish sauce, lemongrass and lime leaves.
Stir well and bring to the boil before reducing to a simmer
and cooking for about 8–10 minutes.

Remove from the heat and let it cool down a little. Discard
the lemongrass and lime leaves before adding to a blender or
using a stick blender to blitz until smooth.

Return to the pan and reheat until piping hot before adding a
squeeze of lime and sprinkling of coriander. Serve.

super-low
cal vegan
soup

PREP 15 minutes	COOK 45 minutes	CALORIES 282

if using gluten-free certified stock

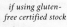

gluten
free

dairy
free

vegan

700 day

spicy bean soup

serves 2

½ tablespoon olive oil
2 garlic cloves, grated
½ teaspoon ground cumin
200g (7oz) canned chopped
  tomatoes
½ tablespoon sun-dried tomato
  paste
300ml (10fl oz) vegetable stock
  (shop-bought or home-made)
½ can (200g/7oz) of red kidney
  beans, drained and rinsed
1 red pepper, cored, deseeded
  and chopped
1 teaspoon cayenne pepper
1 teaspoon dried oregano
sea salt and freshly ground
  pepper

To serve
¼ red onion, sliced
couple of sprigs of fresh
  coriander, chopped

Think of this soup as chilli without the minced beef. Red kidney beans are an excellent source of plant-based protein and fibre, which helps prevent cravings. The lycopene in the concentrated sun-dried tomato paste and canned tomatoes especially protects the body against oxidative stress. It has also been shown to defend the skin against the damaging effects of the sun, all of which add up to a nice little anti-ageing concoction in a bowl. Easy.

Heat the oil in a pan over a medium heat and add the garlic, cumin, chopped tomatoes and sun-dried tomato paste, stirring well for about 2 minutes.

Add the stock and leave to simmer for about 8 minutes.

Pour the stock into a blender or use a stick blender and blitz until smooth. Return to the pan and add the kidney beans, red pepper, cayenne pepper and oregano. Simmer for a further 10–12 minutes, by which time the beans should be warmed through and the pepper should be softening.

Season well and serve with sliced red onion and chopped coriander.

super-low
cal vegan
soup

PREP 8–10 minutes	COOK 25 minutes	CALORIES 162

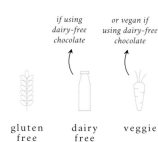

if using
dairy-free
chocolate

or vegan if
using dairy-free
chocolate

gluten
free

dairy
free

veggie

100 day

mini chocolate, matcha & nut butter cups

makes 24

280g (10oz) plain dark chocolate (minimum 70 per cent cocoa), or a dairy-free version, broken into bits
2 teaspoons coconut oil
120g (4¼oz) almond or macadamia nut butter
½–1 teaspoon organic matcha powder, plus extra for sprinkling
2 tablespoons coconut or nut milk (almond, cashew)
1 teaspoon agave syrup, to taste
sea salt

Matcha is rich in powerfully antioxidant catechins, and together with bitter dark chocolate, create a sirtuin-stimulating superbomb dessert. These tiny, bite-sized cups look gorgeous on the plate and will keep in the refrigerator for around 5 days – not that you'll have any left because they're impossible to resist.

Place 24 mini cupcake cases on a tray.

Put a pan over a medium heat with a little water in the bottom and bring it to a simmer. Place a glass bowl over the pan, ensuring the water doesn't touch the bottom of it. Add the chocolate and coconut oil and let them melt, giving them a gentle stir every now and then. When fully melted, remove from the heat. Using a teaspoon, fill the bottom third of each mini cupcake case with some of the melted chocolate mixture (you'll use the rest later). Then put them in the freezer for 10 minutes.

Place the nut butter, matcha, milk and a squeeze of agave syrup in a blender and blitz until smooth. Taste and add more agave syrup if you feel it needs it. Remove the mini cases from the freezer and add 2 teaspoons of the matcha mixture to each one, pressing them down as you go so the tops are smooth. Freeze again for a further 5 minutes.

If the remaining chocolate has started to harden, just gently melt it again using the same method as above. Take the cupcake cases out of the freezer and use a teaspoon to fill them up to the top with the remaining chocolate. Freeze again for 20 minutes. Serve straight from the freezer (or store in the refrigerator) with a sprinkling of matcha and salt on each one.

super-low cal

PREP 15 minutes	COOK 35 minutes	CALORIES 101 per cup

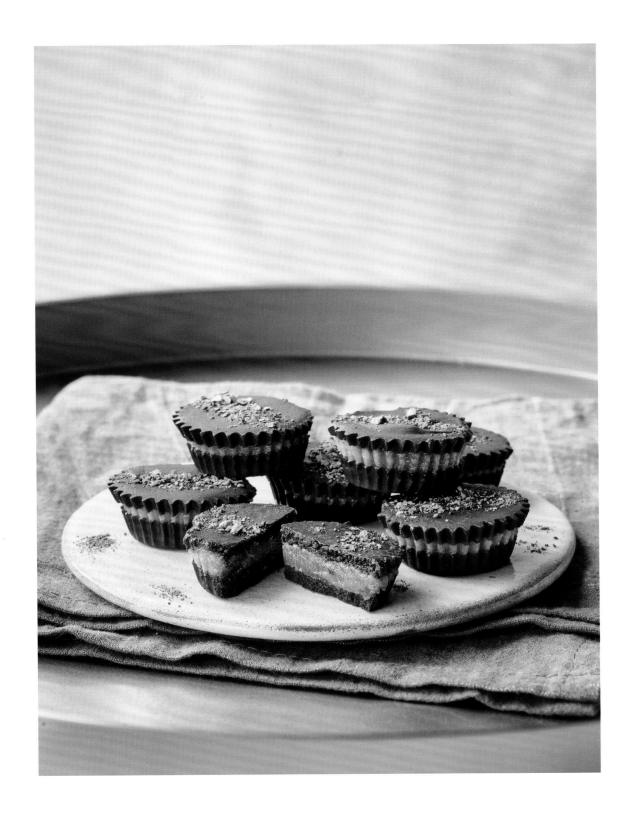

gluten free   veggie

kitchen garden home-made ice cream

each flavour serves 8

for the base
500ml (18fl oz) Greek or natural kefir yogurt
3 tablespoons agave syrup, or more to taste (if required after adding the flavourings)

for raspberry, rosewater and basil flavour
1kg frozen raspberries
1 tablespoon rosewater (less if it's strong)
juice of 1 lemon
purple basil leaves, to serve

for lemon and mint with lime zest flavour
zest and juice of 10 lemons
30g (1oz) mint, leaves removed from stalks, plus extra to serve
lime zest, to serve

for pomegranate, strawberry and thyme flavour
175ml (6fl oz) pure pomegranate juice
400g (14oz) frozen strawberries
leaves of 2 sprigs of thyme, plus extra sprigs to serve

super-low cal

What is life without ice cream? This is the healthy cousin of the traditional sugary version, and it brings all the creamy sweetness with none of the meanness. These recipes are highly adaptable, so throw in whichever fruit you particularly love, adjusting the sweetness according to taste. Adding herbs makes them a little bit sophisticated – and there's nothing wrong with that.

Mix up the base ingredients together in a bowl to form your base.

Place the ingredients for your chosen flavour into a blender and blitz together.

Mix with the base, transfer to a freezerproof container and freeze for 4 hours or overnight.

Remove from the freezer 30 minutes before serving and finish with the basil leaves, lime zest or extra thyme.

PREP	FREEZE	CALORIES PER SCOOP
5 minutes	4 hours or overnight	140 for raspberry and rosewater flavour 95 for lemon and mint flavour 124 for pomegranate & strawberry flavour

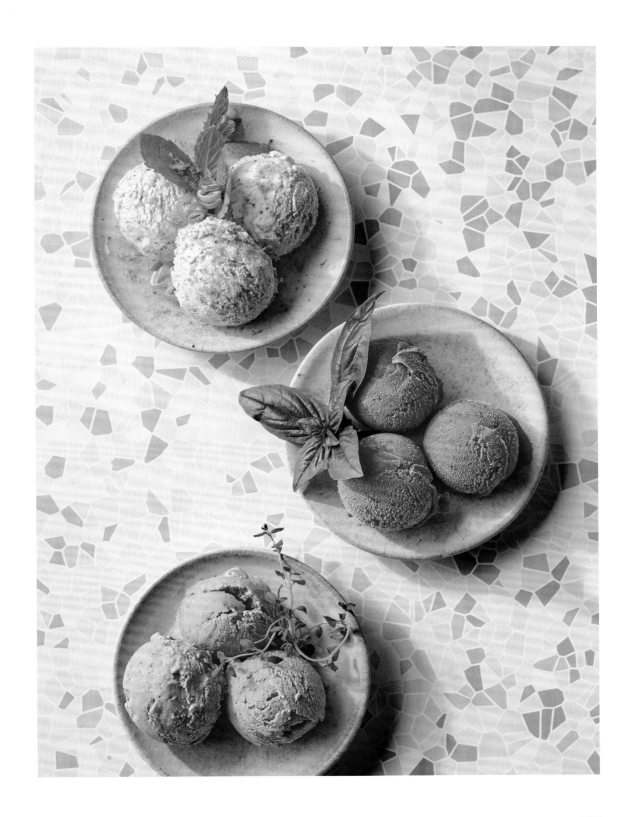

mindful
recipes

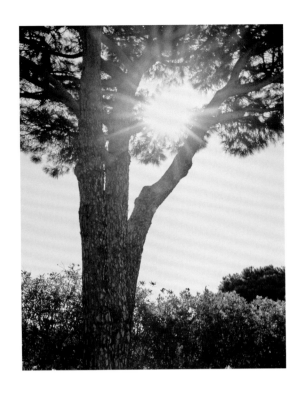
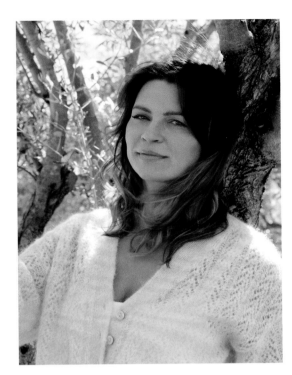
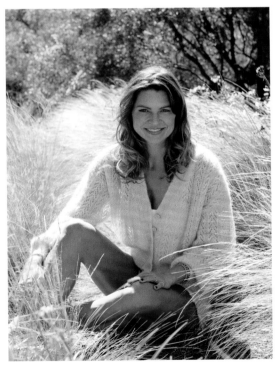
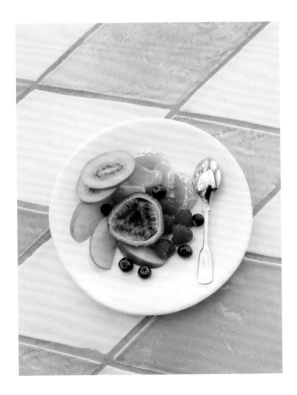

gluten
free

dairy
free

vegan

super-charged banana smoothie

serves 1

1 small banana
200ml (7fl oz) plant-based milk
  (almond, coconut, oat)
2 tablespoons vegan chocolate
  protein powder
2 tablespoons almond butter
  (optional)
2 tablespoons nuts or seeds –
  anything you have at home
½ tablespoon coconut oil
½ teaspoon ground cinnamon
shot of espresso (optional)
squeeze of agave syrup, to
  taste (optional)
sprinkle of cocoa powder
  (optional)

Energy-boosting and highly nutritious, this is a meal on the go – breakfast, snack – whatever works for you. This sweet, chocolatey, protein-packed smoothie is rich in good fats like omega 3 and coconut oil – and coffee lovers can throw in a shot of espresso, which will be balanced out by the good fats and protein content. It's outrageous that this is actually good for you.

Blitz all the ingredients together in a blender until smooth, adding a little water until it has your preferred consistency.

Pour into a flask if you're on the run, or you could serve the smoothie in a teacup if you're at home and you're feeling cute, and finish it with a sprinkling of cocoa powder.

PREP	CALORIES
5 minutes	658 with almond milk
	462 without almond butter

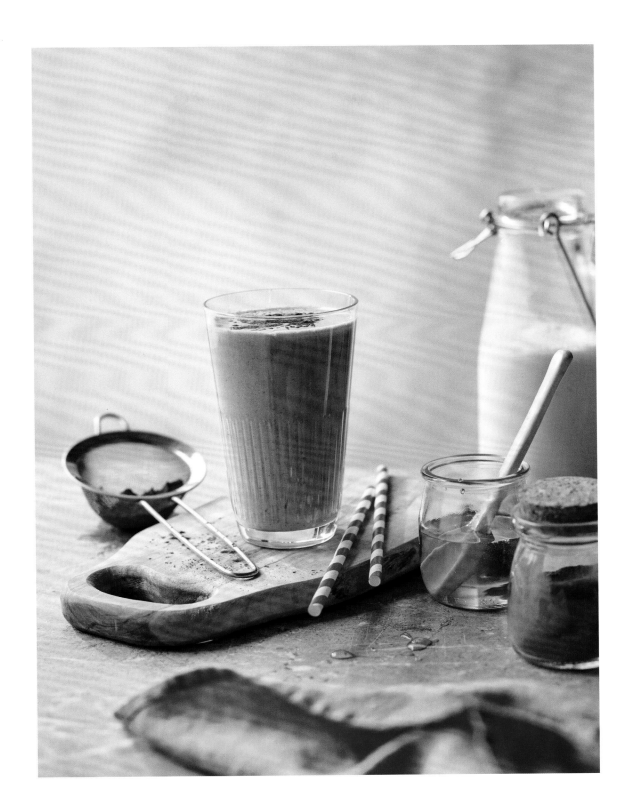

gluten
free

veggie

*if using
gluten-free
certified oats*

Mindful day

golden sunrise bowl

serves 1

2 teaspoons ground turmeric or
8cm (3¼-inch) piece of fresh
turmeric, peeled and grated

2cm (¾-inch) piece of fresh
ginger, peeled and grated

3 tablespoons Greek yogurt or
nut yogurt (coconut, almond)

40g (1½oz) rolled oats (gluten-
free, if preferred)

1 tablespoon nut butter (almond,
cashew, hazelnut)

1 banana, broken into small
pieces

½ mango, peeled, stoned and
roughly chopped

½ teaspoon ground cinnamon

up to 250ml (9fl oz) water

to serve

(optional – add 39 caloriesl)

30g (1oz) pomegranate seeds

40g (1½oz) mango flesh, chopped

1 tablespoon hemp seeds or
flaxseeds

Creamy and delicious. The beauty of this recipe is that
you can make it the night before and then wake up
smiling, knowing that breakfast is ready and waiting
in the refrigerator. Starring alongside turmeric, the
longevity and anti-inflammatory superhero, the oats
are highly nutritious and a fantastic source of fibre –
including beta-glucans, the soluble fibre that stimulates
the immune system and absorbs cholesterol.

Add all the ingredients to a blender and blitz until smooth,
adding splashes of water along the way to make it the
consistency of your choice (I like it quite thick, so don't tend
to add too much water, and no more than 250ml/9fl oz).

Serve in a bowl with pomegranate seeds, mango and hemp
or flax seeds sprinkled over, if you like.

PREP	CALORIES
10 minutes	236 with Greek yogurt
	460 with nut yogurt

if using gluten-free certified oats and baking powder

gluten
free

dairy
free

vegan

Mindful day

chewy quinoa cookies

makes 14

1 tablespoon ground flaxseeds
1 tablespoon chia seeds
5 tablespoons warm water
90g (3¼oz) oat flour (gluten-
   free, if preferred)
80g (3oz) rolled oats (gluten-
   free, if preferred)
½ teaspoon baking powder
   (gluten-free, if preferred)
½ teaspoon ground cinnamon
½ teaspoon ground nutmeg
½ teaspoon ground ginger
90g (3¼oz) precooked quinoa
pinch of sea salt
2 carrots, grated
70g (2½oz) mixed seeds
   (sunflower, pumpkin, hemp)
60g (2¼oz) dried goji berries
zest of ½ lemon
110g (4oz) nut butter (cashew,
   almond)
5 tablespoons coconut oil,
   melted
5 tablespoons agave syrup

There are few cookies in life you can tuck into for breakfast without raising suspicion that you've got a hangover, but these are the exception. From the multitude of omega 3-packed seeds to fibre-rich oats, which are champions of a healthy digestion, these delicious, chewy cookies have a glorious texture thanks to the blend of sweet carrots, goji berries and coconut oil. And again, they can live beyond the realms of breakfast as a snack at any time of the day.

Preheat the oven to 200°C (400°F), Gas Mark 6 and line a large baking tray with nonstick baking paper.

Add the flaxseeds and chia seeds to a bowl with the warm water and mix. You want them to become a bit gloopy, so leave them while you prepare the other ingredients.

Add the oat flour, rolled oats, baking powder, cinnamon, nutmeg, ginger, quinoa and pinch of salt to a separate bowl, mixing well. Then add the carrots, mixed seeds, goji berries and lemon zest and mix until thoroughly coated.

In another bowl, combine the nut butter, coconut oil and agave syrup, mixing well before adding the water, flax and chia mixture. Add this wet mixture to the dry ingredients and thoroughly mix.

Using a tablespoon, drop spoonfuls of the mixture onto the tray, making sure there is space between each one. Bake in the oven for about 16–18 minutes or until golden. Remove from the oven and cool slightly, then transfer to a wire rack to cool completely. The cookies can then happily live in an airtight container for 1 week.

PREP 15 minutes	COOK 20 minutes	CALORIES 218 per cookie

gluten
free

dairy
free

chilli-salt salmon

serves 2

2 200g (7oz) salmon fillets, skin
removed
1 tablespoon sea salt
1 teaspoon chilli flakes
½ teaspoon garlic powder
1 teaspoon lemon zest
lemon juice, to serve (optional)

for the chopped salad

¼ cucumber, chopped into 1cm
(½-inch) cubes
2 carrots, grated
2 celery sticks, chopped into
small pieces
10 cherry tomatoes, halved
1 yellow pepper, cored, deseeded
and chopped into small pieces
¼ red onion, finely chopped
juice of ½ lime
1 Little Gem lettuce, chopped
15g (½oz) pumpkin seeds

for the dressing

1 teaspoon Dijon mustard
1 tablespoon balsamic vinegar
2 tablespoons extra virgin olive
oil
sea salt and freshly ground
pepper

Salmon is the ultimate brain food. It's also good for glowing skin and healthy hair – so you'll not only finish lunch probably more intelligent than when you started, you'll undoubtedly look fabulous too. Salmon can sometimes be a bit samey, so this recipe mixes things up a little with a delicious chilli and salt blend. It's super-quick, too, which also gives it extra house points. Oh, and don't throw away the omega-3-rich salmon skin. It's delicious fried up on its own and eaten with a sprinkling of salt.

Cut each salmon fillet in half so that you have four squarish pieces. Mix the sea salt, chilli flakes, garlic powder and lemon zest together in a small bowl and sprinkle over the fish. Refrigerate for 1 hour.

Preheat the oven to 240°C (475°F), Gas Mark 9 and line a baking tray with foil or nonstick baking paper.

Place the marinated salmon on the lined tray. Bake for 10 minutes or until it has cooked through.

While the salmon is cooking, add all the chopped salad ingredients to a bowl. Whisk the dressing ingredients together in a small jug and pour over the salad ingredients, mixing everything together.

Serve the salad with the cooked salmon – and add a squeeze of lemon, if so inclined.

PREP	CHILL	COOK	CALORIES
20 minutes	1 hour	10 minutes	478

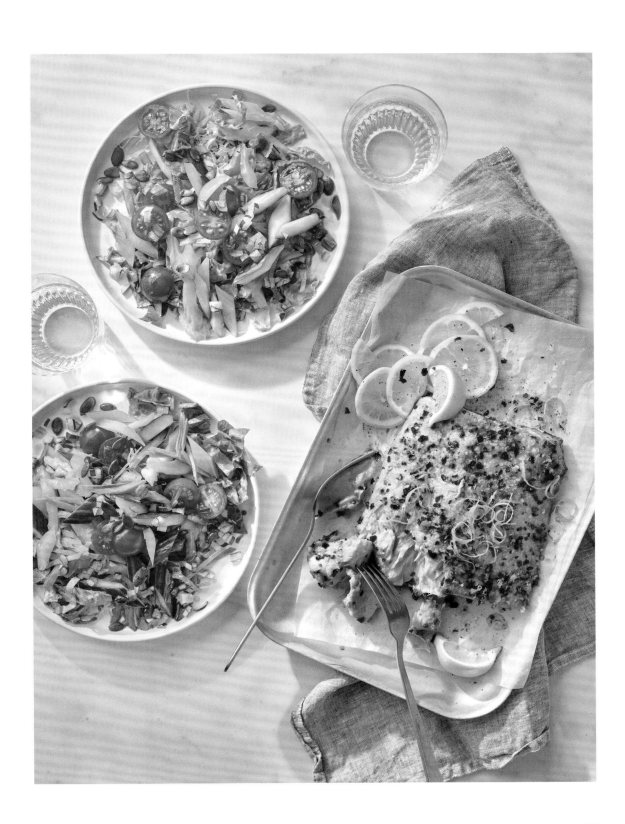

dairy free   vegan

vegan burritos

serves 4

200g (7oz) can of sweetcorn, drained
½ can (200g/7oz) of black beans, drained and rinsed
1 yellow or orange pepper, cored, deseeded and chopped
¼ red onion, finely chopped
1 red chilli, deseeded and sliced
100g (3½oz) baby spinach leaves
20g (¾oz) fresh coriander leaves, roughly chopped
½ teaspoon smoked paprika
flesh of ½ ripe avocado, mushed with a fork
4 large wholemeal tortillas
100g (3½oz) lettuce of your choice, shredded
100g (3½oz) precooked brown rice

If I'm being brutally honest, this is really a go-to recipe for hangovers. Filling and nutritious, it's exactly the kind of restorative, comfort food that will help even the sorest of heads on the road to recovery. The good news is you don't need to have had a heavy night to tuck into one of these Tex-Mex favourites. They're great on the go, too – just wrap them in foil, grab your keys and don't look back.

Add the sweetcorn, black beans, pepper, onion, chilli, spinach, coriander, smoked paprika and avocado to a largish bowl and mix everything together.

Place a tortilla on a plate and add some of the lettuce and rice to the centre of it. Then add some of the burrito mixture. How much will depend on the size of your tortillas, but don't go too mad as you don't want it to burst out of the tortilla when you wrap it.

Fold over the sides as if you are wrapping a parcel and then wrap the whole thing in foil. Cut it in half with a sharp knife and fold back a little of the foil so you can start munching on it. Repeat to make the rest of the burritos.

PREP 20 minutes	CALORIES 337

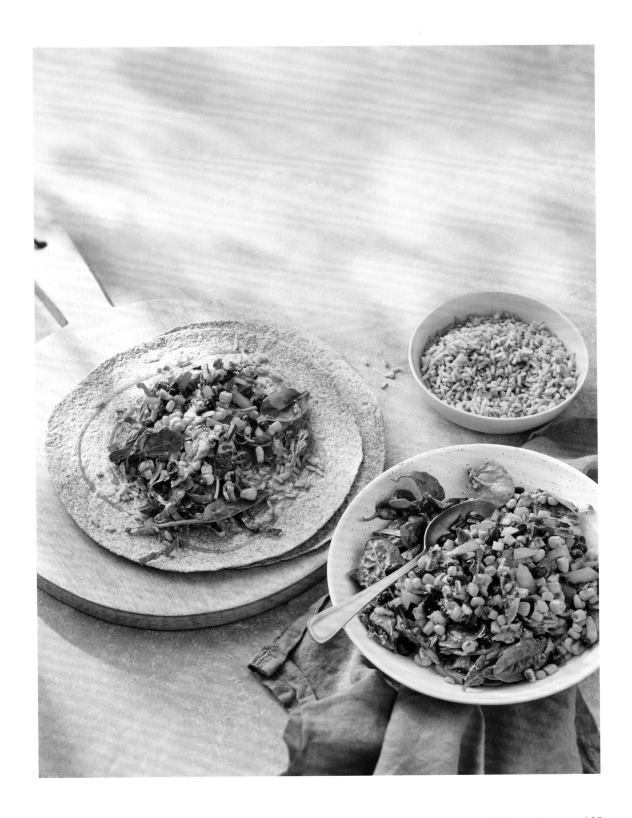

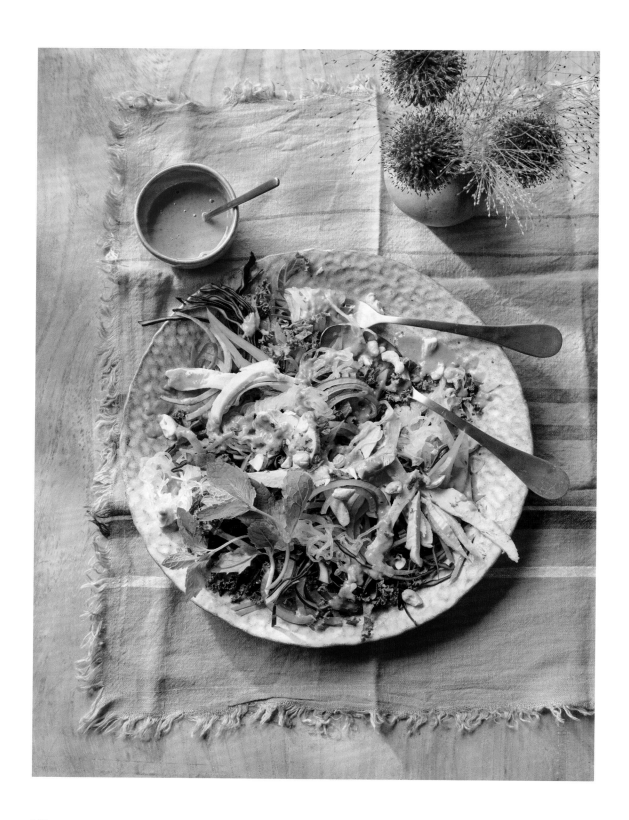

gluten
free

dairy
free

chicken satay noodle salad

serves 4

2 organic or free-range chicken
  breasts
1 tablespoon rapeseed oil
200g (7oz) glass noodles or zero-
  calorie konjac noodles
handful of kale (approx.
  20g/¾oz), stalks removed and
  thinly sliced
½ small red cabbage, thinly
  sliced
2 carrots, grated
1 yellow pepper, cored, deseeded
  and thinly sliced
¼ red onion, thinly sliced
1 red chilli, deseeded and thinly
  sliced
small handful of mint, torn
20g (¾oz) cashew nuts, halved
  (reserve 4, chopped, to serve)
sea salt and freshly ground
  pepper

for the dressing

2 tablespoons crunchy nut butter
  (cashew, peanut)
1 tablespoon tamari
2 teaspoons agave syrup
2cm (¾-inch) piece of fresh
  ginger, peeled and grated
½ garlic clove, grated
¼ teaspoon cayenne pepper
juice of 2 limes

Chicken satay. YUM. This is a take on the Southeast Asian classic, but with a considerably healthier twist. Think lots of shredded raw vegetables, plenty of herbs, the crunch of the odd cashew nut and satay sauce reimagined with the heat of cayenne pepper and ginger, but just as delicious. Like a Chinese takeaway, but not as you know it.

Place the chicken breasts between two sheets of nonstick baking paper and bash with a rolling pin until about 1cm (½ inch) thick. Season each side well.

Heat the oil in a large pan over a medium heat and fry the chicken breasts until golden and cooked through – about 3 minutes on each side. Let them cool a little and then cut them into thin slices.

Prepare the noodles according to the packet instructions – if this involves soaking them in boiling water, rinse them in cold water once they're soft and then drain well.

Add the kale, cabbage, carrots, pepper, onion, chilli, mint and cashew nuts to a large bowl before adding the cooled noodles and warm chicken. Mix well.

Whisk the dressing ingredients together in a small bowl and pour over the chicken salad and noodles. Serve with the reserved chopped cashew nuts sprinkled on top.

PREP 20 minutes	COOK 10 minutes	CALORIES 328 with glass noodles 255 with zero-calorie konjac noodles

dairy
free

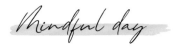

healthy tuna burger

serves 4

500g (1lb 2oz) fresh, sustainably
  sourced tuna steak, chopped
  into small pieces
small handful of fresh coriander
  leaves (approx. 20g/¾oz),
  chopped
small handful of Thai basil
  leaves (approx. 20g/¾oz), torn
1 garlic clove, grated
2cm (¾-inch) piece of fresh
  ginger, peeled and grated
1 tablespoon white miso paste
1 tablespoon tamari
1 tablespoon olive oil
1 red chilli, deseeded and finely
  chopped
zest and juice of 1 lime, plus
  extra lime juice, to serve
4 wholemeal pittas
handful of rocket
flesh of 1 ripe avocado, sliced
1 red pepper, cored, deseeded
  and thinly sliced
sea salt and freshly ground
  pepper
4 tablespoons mayonnaise, to
  serve (with an optional squeeze
  of sriracha, yuzu or lime)

This is a great family-friendly recipe and makes a delicious addition to a barbecue lunch in the summer. Tuna is low in calories, high in protein and a spectacular source of omega 3 and vitamin D. Say hello to healthier bones and a stronger immune system. Wholemeal pitta instead of an evil processed burger bun is another way to up the health stakes, while getting creative with mayonnaise will make this even more sophisticated and interesting (especially for grown-ups): try adding some sriracha or yuzu. Delicious.

Place the tuna, coriander, Thai basil, garlic, ginger, miso, tamari, half the olive oil, the chilli and the lime zest and juice in a bowl, seasoning well with salt and pepper. Mix well and shape into four burger patties. Cover and refrigerate for about 30 minutes.

Preheat the oven to 200°C (400°F), Gas Mark 6, and warm the pittas in it for 5 minutes.

While that's going on, heat the other half of the olive oil in a frying pan over a highish heat and add the burgers. Cook them for about 2 minutes per side if you like them pink on the inside, or longer if you prefer more colour.

Halve the warm pittas and add the rocket, avocado, pepper and tuna burgers. Serve with a hearty dollop of mayonnaise and an optional squeeze of sriracha, yuzu or spritz of lime.

PREP	COOK	CHILL	CALORIES
15 minutes	5 minutes	30 minutes	480

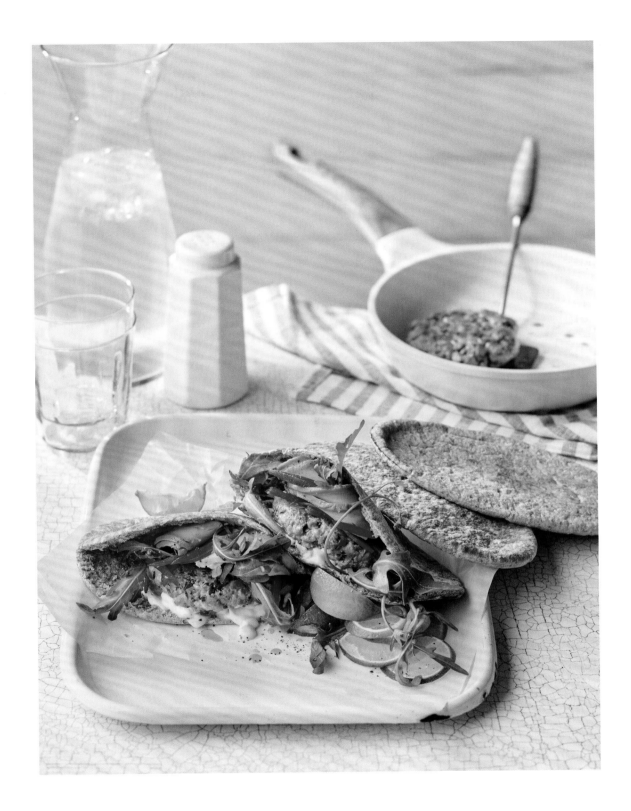

if using gluten-free certified rotis

gluten
free

dairy
free

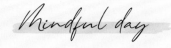

chicken & red lentil saag

serves 4

1 onion, finely chopped
4cm (1½-inch) piece of fresh
  ginger, peeled and grated
2 red chillies, deseeded and
  finely chopped
2 garlic cloves, grated
1 tablespoon coconut oil
1 teaspoon coriander seeds,
  crushed
1 teaspoon ground turmeric
1 teaspoon ground cumin
1 teaspoon garam masala
2 organic or free-range chicken
  breasts (approx. 350g/12oz),
  skin removed and cut into
  roughly 4cm/1½-inch pieces
180g (6½oz) dried red split
  lentils
400g (14oz) can of chopped
  tomatoes
300g (10½oz) spinach
brown rice, quinoa or wholemeal
  rotis, to serve (optional)

This Indian-inspired dish is an aromatic powerhouse of goodness. Anti-inflammatory turmeric and ginger work beautifully with all the spices to make this a warming, healthy delight. Vegetarians and vegans can remove the chicken, but maintain a protein punch, thanks to the lentils. Definitely a crowd pleaser.

Add the onion, ginger, red chillies and garlic to a pestle and mortar and grind them into a paste.

Heat the coconut oil in a large pan over a medium heat and add the paste. Cook for a couple of minutes, then add the spices, cooking for another minute or so until lovely and fragrant. Add the chicken, stirring well so that it's coated with the spicy paste. Cook for 5 minutes.

Add the lentils and tomatoes next. Fill the empty can of tomatoes with water, slosh it around and add that to the mixture. Stir well. Turn down the heat and leave it to simmer gently for about 30 minutes or until the lentils are tender.

At the very end, stir in the spinach and make sure it has wilted. Serve with brown rice, quinoa or wholemeal rotis.

PREP 15 minutes	COOK 35 minutes	CALORIES 317

gluten
free

dairy
free

no-bread turkey wraps

serves 2

1 tablespoon rapeseed oil
250g (9oz) minced turkey
½ teaspoon Chinese five spice
1 large carrot, grated
2 spring onions, thinly sliced
50g (1¾oz) sugar snap peas,
    thinly sliced on the diagonal
1 garlic clove, grated
2cm (¾-inch) piece of fresh
    ginger, peeled and grated
2 tablespoons hoisin sauce
½ tablespoon sriracha
80g (3oz) lettuce leaves,
    (Romaine, butterhead, iceberg,
    Little Gem)
1 red chilli, deseeded and thinly
    sliced (optional)
sea salt and freshly ground
    pepper

Turkey doesn't need to be consigned to one time of the year. It's low in fat, higher in protein than chicken and contains plenty of tryptophan and magnesium – essential nutrients that make all the difference when it comes to a good night's sleep – but don't worry, you won't fall asleep at the table with your face in a lettuce wrap. Hopefully.

Heat the oil in a frying pan over a medium-high heat and add the turkey, Chinese five spice and some seasoning. Fry until the meat is cooked through and has some colour – about 4–5 minutes.

Remove the pan from the heat and transfer the turkey to a bowl. Now add the carrot, spring onions, sugar snap peas, garlic and ginger, combining well.

Mix the hoisin and sriracha in a small bowl.

Lay out the lettuce leaves on a plate and spoon some turkey mixture into each one. Drizzle over the hoisin and sriracha sauce and add a few slices of red chilli to each, if you want a little kick.

PREP 10 minutes	COOK 5 minutes	CALORIES 336

gluten
free

dairy
free

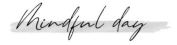

wild rice, salmon & kimchi salad

serves 4

100g (3½oz) wild rice mix
1 large salmon fillet (approx.
   170g/6oz), skin removed
1 tablespoon tamari
zest and juice of ½ lemon, plus
   extra juice, to taste
1 garlic clove, grated
2 tablespoons kimchi
¼ cucumber, chopped
8 cherry tomatoes, halved
small bunch of flat-leaf parsley,
   chopped
1 tablespoon sprouted grains or
   seeds (alfalfa, broccoli, kale,
   lentil, chickpea)
sea salt and freshly ground
   pepper
2 teaspoons extra virgin olive
   oil, to serve (optional)

Chewy and almost slightly nutty in flavour, wild rice is a fantastic source of fibre and will help keep energy levels nice and balanced by keeping you fuller for longer. It also helps support good bacteria in the digestive system, which along with the probiotic power of kimchi, makes it an amazing dish to keep returning to if healthy weight loss is your goal. For those not confident cooking rice, precooked packages are really excellent these days – I'm definitely a fan.

Preheat the oven to 200°C (400°F), Gas Mark 6 and line a baking tray with a large piece of foil.

Cook the rice according to the packet instructions.

While that's bubbling away, put the salmon in the centre of the lined tray. Add the tamari, lemon zest and juice and garlic, making sure the salmon is nicely covered. Season well, then close up the foil to form a loose bag around the salmon – make sure the seal is nice and secure as you don't want any steam to escape. Bake for 20 minutes or until it's cooked through. Then set aside to cool until about room temperature.

Place the kimchi, cucumber, tomatoes, parsley and sprouted grains or seeds in a bowl with the rice and mix together. Then flake the salmon with your fingers and add to the bowl. Mix gently and transfer to plates, perhaps with another pinch of salt, grind of pepper, squeeze of lemon and the optional extra virgin olive oil. You may now tuck in.

PREP	COOK	CALORIES
10 minutes	25 minutes	319 (without extra virgin olive oil)
		399 (with extra virgin olive oil)

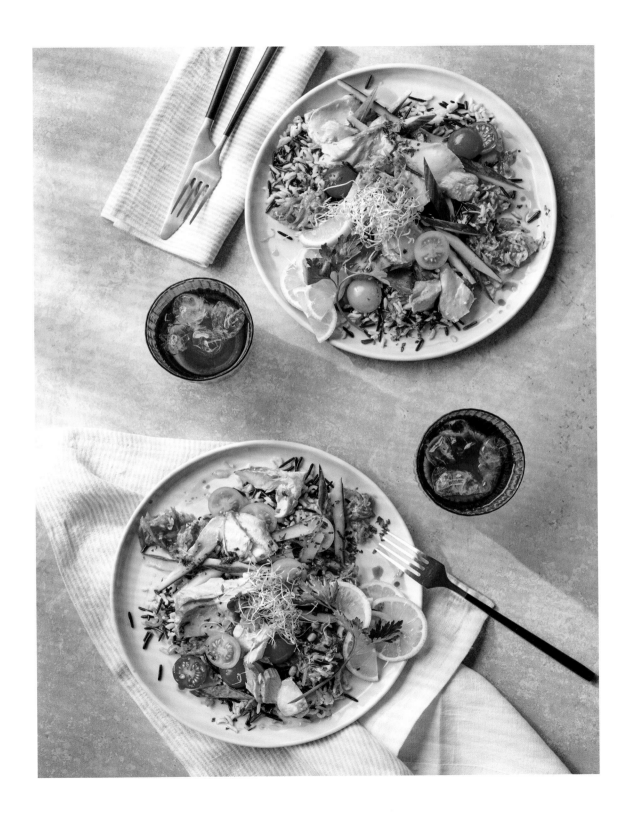

dairy
free

vegan

avocado & spicy roasted chickpeas on toast

serves 2

for the chickpeas

½ can (200g/7oz) of chickpeas,
   drained and rinsed
½ tablespoon olive oil
½ teaspoon cayenne pepper
½ teaspoon garlic powder
¼ teaspoon ground turmeric
sea salt and freshly ground
   pepper

for the tahini dressing

40g (1½oz) smooth tahini
1 garlic clove, grated
½ teaspoon sesame oil
½ tablespoon extra virgin olive
   oil
1 tablespoon lemon juice
boiled water, for consistency
   (optional)
sea salt and freshly ground
   pepper

for the avocado toast

2 slices of grain-heavy bread
   (rye, pumpernickel, mixed seed
   loaf), toasted
flesh of 1 ripe avocado
1 spring onion, sliced
juice of ½ lime
sea salt and freshly ground
   pepper

There's no time of day these spicy, crunchy chickpeas on toast won't work: a hearty breakfast, a mid-morning snack, a light lunch or supper. The mixture of protein and healthy fats from the avocado is lovely and filling. Avocados are surprisingly high in fibre, so this winning combination helps the body feel satisfied, plus it's a particularly good recipe for all you longevity fans. See you in 100 years!

Preheat the oven to 220°C (425°F), Gas Mark 7.

Pat the chickpeas dry with a tea towel and then place in a bowl with the olive oil, cayenne pepper, garlic powder, turmeric and seasoning, mixing well to ensure the chickpeas are thoroughly coated. Spread the mixture out on a baking tray and roast for 25–30 minutes or until golden and crispy. Then set aside to cool a little.

Place the tahini, garlic, sesame oil, extra virgin olive oil, lemon juice and seasoning in a bowl and whisk together to make the dressing. Add a splash of boiled water if it's too thick, but do it incrementally so you don't end up with something too thin.

Toast the bread and while it's toasting, mash the avocado with a fork in a bowl and add most of the spring onion, the lime juice and some seasoning. Let the toast cool a little before spooning on the avocado mixture.

Top with the roasted chickpeas, drizzle over the tahini dressing and add the remaining spring onion.

PREP 10 minutes	COOK 25–30 minutes	CALORIES 561

gluten
free

veggie

angelic eggs

serves 6

6 organic or free-range eggs, at
    room temperature
1 tablespoon mayonnaise
2 tablespoons Greek or live
    natural yogurt
½ teaspoon Dijon mustard
½ teaspoon horseradish
sea salt and freshly ground
    pepper

for the toppings

chopped chives
celery salt
smoked paprika

The egg recipe on this page and overleaf make glorious canapés and afternoon snacks, if you're the kind of person who really goes for it when it comes to afternoon snacks, especially if they're just for you. In fact, if you make both recipes together, they would work as a light starter at a dinner party. I'm so here for eggs and their vitamin B content. Bring me more eggs so I can dance all night.

Bring a pan of water to the boil. Carefully add the eggs and simmer gently for 8 minutes to hard boil. Carefully remove the eggs and hold them under cold running water to cool. Once they're cool enough to handle, peel them and cut them in half. Remove the yolks and reserve the yolks and whites separately.

Place the reserved yolks in a blender with the mayonnaise, yogurt, mustard and horseradish and blitz until smooth. Season to taste.

Spoon or pipe the mixture into the reserved egg white halves and sprinkle with any or all of the suggested toppings before serving.

PREP 15 minutes	COOK 10 minutes	CALORIES 92

gluten
free

eggs with prawns & celery

serves 6

6 organic or free-range eggs, at
  room temperature
100g (3½oz) cooked peeled
  prawns, chopped
½ celery stick, finely chopped
¼ cucumber, finely chopped
2 tablespoons mayonnaise
2 tablespoons Greek or live
  natural yogurt
1 teaspoon chilli flakes
squeeze of lemon juice
sea salt and freshly ground
  pepper
flat-leaf parsley sprigs, to serve

The second of our egg snack recipes brings prawns to the party. Mixed together with refreshing cucumber and crunchy celery, you can keep them in the fridge and graze on them throughout the day. In fact, if you want to reduce the calorie content even further, remove the yolks and stuff them with this delicious mixture.

Bring a pan of water to the boil. Carefully add the eggs and simmer gently for 8 minutes to hard boil. Carefully remove the eggs and hold them under cold running water to cool. Once they're cool enough to handle, peel them and cut them in half.

Place the prawns, celery, cucumber, mayonnaise, yogurt, chilli flakes, lemon juice and some seasoning in a bowl and mix well.

Using a teaspoon, add some prawn mixture on top of each egg. Sprinkle with chopped parsley and serve.

| PREP 15 minutes | COOK 10 minutes | CALORIES 171 |

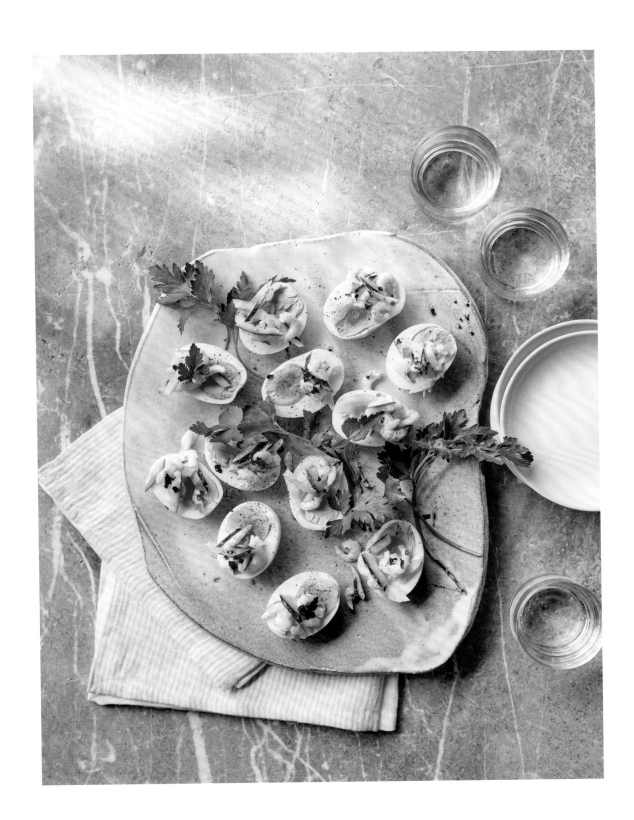

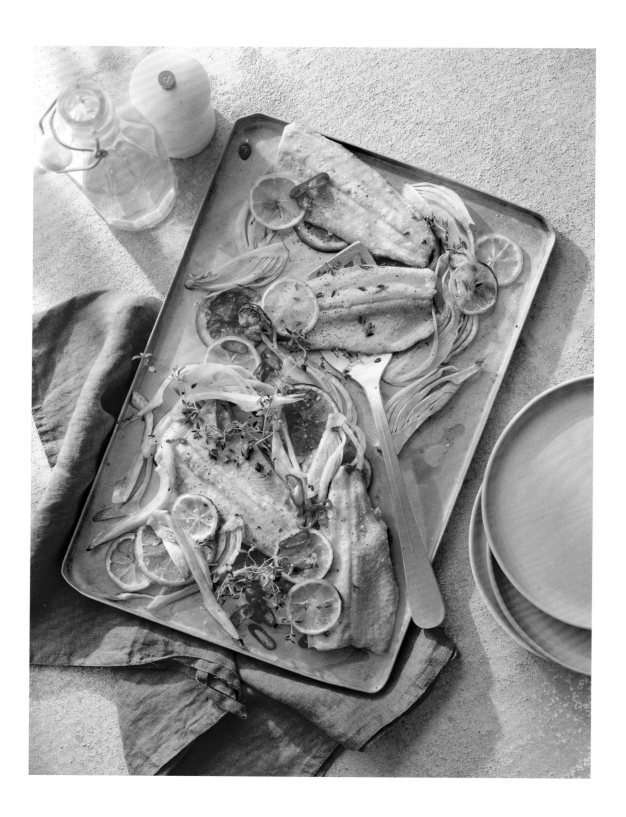

gluten
free

dairy
free

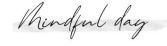

rainbow trout & citrus salad

serves 4

1 small fennel bulb, thinly sliced

1 lemon, thinly sliced, plus
  lemon juice, to taste

1 blood orange, thinly sliced

1 red chilli, deseeded and thinly
  sliced

4 rainbow trout fillets (approx.
  130g/4½oz each)

leaves of 1 small sprig of thyme

2 tablespoons olive oil

sea salt and freshly ground
  pepper

While it might feel like it lives in the shadow of salmon, trout is a delicious, slightly lighter version of its more famous cousin, and just as full of anti-ageing and anti-inflammatory omega 3 and selenium. It's also incredibly high in vitamin D, which is essential for a healthy immune system. Fennel is, of course, very good for digestion, plus it adds a subtle aniseed element to this dish alongside the bright zing of the citrus. The perfect sharing platter for a brunch or light lunch.

Preheat the oven to 200°C (400°F), Gas Mark 6.

Put the fennel, lemon, blood orange and chilli in a shallow roasting tin. Place the trout fillets on top, season well, scatter over the thyme leaves and douse them with the oil. Roast for about 12 minutes or until the fish is cooked through.

Transfer the fish, fennel, citrus slices and chilli slices to a large sharing platter and pour over any juices, adding an extra spritz of lemon if the mood takes you.

PREP 10 minutes	COOK 15 minutes	CALORIES 247

gluten
free

dairy
free

vegan

mini carrot cake bites

makes 12 balls

80g (3oz) walnuts
½ teaspoon ground ginger
½ teaspoon ground cinnamon
¼ teaspoon ground nutmeg
8 soft Medjool dates, pitted
2 carrots, roughly chopped
1 tablespoon agave syrup
pinch of sea salt
50g (1¾oz) ground almonds

Okay, so perhaps some of you hate me right now because I made you eat broth for two weeks. (You wait – the moment someone asks for ID when you're buying a bottle of wine will make it worth it.) Here's a little reward – these delicious little bites are packed full of spices and plenty of protein, which makes them perfect for mid-morning snacks or even just breakfast, because why not?

Place the walnuts, ginger, cinnamon, nutmeg, dates, carrots, agave syrup and salt in a blender and blitz. You want the mixture to be combined and sticky. If it's looking a bit dry, add a splash of water. Refrigerate for about 20 minutes so that it solidifies a little.

Spoon out the mixture and roll into smooth balls in your hands, roughly 3cm (1¼ inches) in size. Sprinkle the ground almonds on a plate and roll the balls through it so they are coated. They'll keep in an airtight container in the refrigerator for up to 5 days, so dip in any time you need a quick sweet treat.

PREP 10 minutes	CALORIES 120 per ball

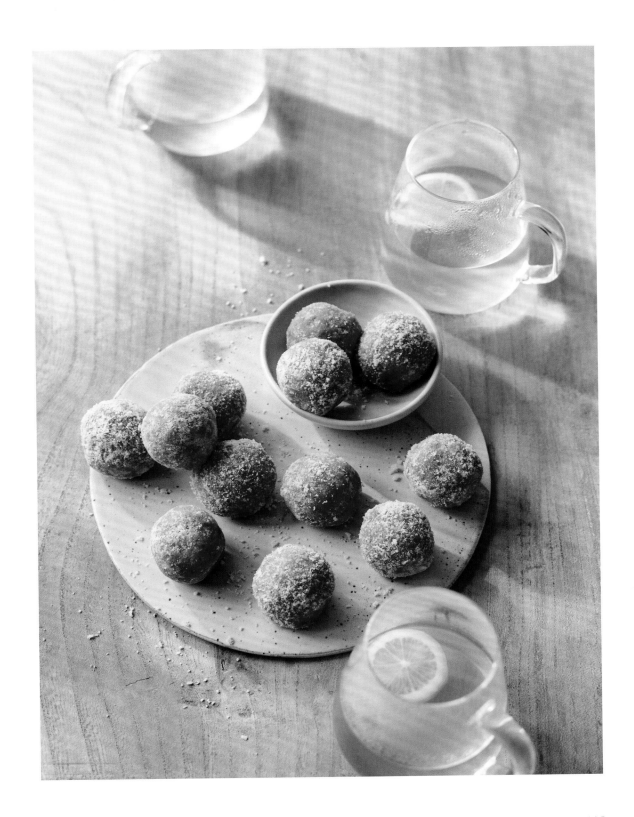

index

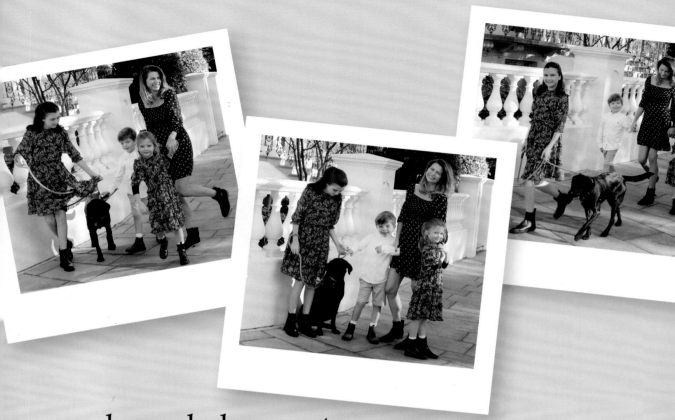

acknowledgements

And now to all the people I need to thank for helping me realise the dream of this second book. I am repaying you with the gift of eternal youth.

To my husband, David – I don't know where I'd be without your support. Probably not the founder of a company or a best-selling author (I may or may not have mentioned that). Or the mother of three children, one dog, two cats, two guinea pigs and four tortoises. Maia, Iris and Caspar – Mummy didn't abandon you, she just wrote a second book. Don't worry, I'm back now (until the third book). Mum, Dad and both my grannies, thank you for being my number one fans. I love you all very much and couldn't do any of it without you.

My lovely, talented, patient and hilarious Clare Bennett. You are absolutely integral to this process of book writing – I truly love the books that we have created. I cherish our friendship, which makes the hours and hours (and hours) of calls a joy.

My agent, Adrian Sington, the team at Kyle Books – Judith Hannam, Isabel Jessop and Claire Rogers – thank you for everything you've done to help make this book happen. Thank you also to the brilliant

GP nutrition team for packaging my advice into pills and powders, and putting words into action.

Many thanks to Max and Ros Dundas and all the Dundas Lifestyle team, and Victoria Scales and Charlotte Sanders at Octopus for everything you'll do to help make it sell (fingers crossed!!!!). Also to Nikki Dupin and Kate Whitaker for making the book look beautiful. And special thanks to the amazing and brilliant Kate Martin and Arabella Boyce for me making me look beautiful.

To my friends – you are still around despite me always being busy and unavailable, which I cannot thank you enough for. You have backed me all the way in everything I do and that means the world to me.

And to my clients – you're my constant inspiration and teachers. Being part of the journey to you feeling your best is a privilege (I told you, you didn't need sugar). And to my followers, old and new – we are all part of a growing community and your questions keep the conversation going. I am so humbled by your kind messages. You're the reason why I do this job.